NUTRITION

AT YOUR FINGERTIPS

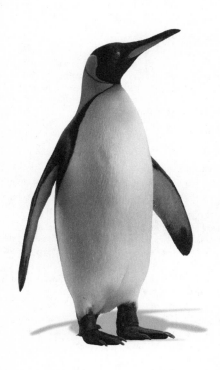

Elisa Zied, MS, RD, CDN

ALPHA

A member of Penguin Group (USA) Inc.

To my older son Spencer for inspiring me to write a third book, to my younger son Eli for following in my footsteps with his amazing Back to Africa books, to my true love Brian for his unwavering love and support, and to my wonderful parents.

ALPHA BOOKS

Published by the Penguin Group

Penguin Group (USA) Inc., 375 Hudson Street, New York, New York 10014, USA

Penguin Group (Canada), 90 Eglinton Avenue East, Suite 700, Toronto, Ontario M4P 2Y3, Canada (a division of Pearson Penguin Canada Inc.)

Penguin Books Ltd., 80 Strand, London WC2R 0RL, England

Penguin Ireland, 25 St. Stephen's Green, Dublin 2, Ireland (a division of Penguin Books Ltd.)

Penguin Group (Australia), 250 Camberwell Road, Camberwell, Victoria 3124, Australia (a division of Pearson Australia Group Pty. Ltd.)

Penguin Books India Pvt. Ltd., 11 Community Centre, Panchsheel Park, New Delhi—110 017, India

Penguin Group (NZ), 67 Apollo Drive, Rosedale, North Shore, Auckland 1311, New Zealand (a division of Pearson New Zealand Ltd.)

Penguin Books (South Africa) (Pty.) Ltd., 24 Sturdee Avenue, Rosebank, Johannesburg 2196, South Africa

Penguin Books Ltd., Registered Offices: 80 Strand, London WC2R 0RL, England

Copyright © 2009 Elisa Zied and The Stonesong Press

International Standard Book Number: 978-1-59257-902-0
Library of Congress Catalog Card Number: 2009926596

11 10 09   8 7 6 5 4 3 2 1

Interpretation of the printing code: The rightmost number of the first series of numbers is the year of the book's printing; the rightmost number of the second series of numbers is the number of the book's printing. For example, a printing code of 09-1 shows that the first printing occurred in 2009.

Printed in the United States of America

Note: This publication contains the opinions and ideas of its author. It is intended to provide helpful and informative material on the subject matter covered. It is sold with the understanding that the author and publisher are not engaged in rendering professional services in the book. If the reader requires personal assistance or advice, a competent professional should be consulted.

The author and publisher specifically disclaim any responsibility for any liability, loss, or risk, personal or otherwise, which is incurred as a consequence, directly or indirectly, of the use and application of any of the contents of this book.

Most Alpha books are available at special quantity discounts for bulk purchases for sales promotions, premiums, fund-raising, or educational use. Special books, or book excerpts, can also be created to fit specific needs.

For details, write: Special Markets, Alpha Books, 375 Hudson Street, New York, NY 10014.

Publisher: **Marie Butler-Knight**
Editorial Director: **Mike Sanders**
Senior Managing Editor: **Billy Fields**
Senior Acquisitions Editor: **Paul Dinas**
Development Editor: **Ginny Bess Munroe**
Senior Production Editor: **Janette Lynn**
Copy Editor: **Megan Wade**

Cover/Book Designer: **Kurt Owens**
Indexer: **Celia McCoy**
Layout: **Brian Massey**
Proofreader: **John Etchison**

CONTENTS

INTRODUCTION

Nutrition is more of a hot topic in the media and on people's minds than ever before. Not a day goes by when there aren't countless articles written in magazines, newspapers, and on the Web or television news segments aired that focus on some aspect of nutrition. While interest in nutrition is widespread, many people don't know whether the information comes from a reliable source, is based on sound science, or can be applied to their lives in a practical way.

Nutrition at Your Fingertips provides all the information you need to understand the science of nutrition and incorporate healthful nutrition practices into your life and that of your family. Whether you have always taken an interest in and have a general understanding of nutrition or you're new to the world of nutrition, this book is organized to help you find accurate, easy-to-understand information you're looking for quickly and easily.

How This Book Is Organized

Nutrition at Your Fingertips is organized like this. First, the key nutrients your body needs and that are found in the diet, including carbohydrate, fat, protein, vitamins, and minerals, are covered. Then I show you how to determine your daily calorie needs and create your own daily eating plan no matter your age or stage of life. Whether you're trying to manage your weight, a diet-related medical condition, or a food allergy or sensitivity, you'll find how-to nutrition strategies throughout the book. The book also includes information to help you navigate the aisles of your local grocery store in a more informed way, read and understand food labels, and ultimately fill your cart with the most delicious and healthful items from all the basic food categories.

The **SEE ALSO** references sprinkled throughout the chapters help you easily locate cross-referenced material in other chapters.

◀ *SEE ALSO 1.1, "Functions of Carbohydrates"* ▶

WORDS TO GO . . . *WORDS TO GO . . . WORDS TO GO*

Words to Go appear at the end of each chapter to give you quick and readily available definitions to help you better understand the material covered in that chapter.

Here's a brief description of each of the chapters:

Chapter 1, "Carbohydrates": This chapter explains the functions of carbohydrates, covers the various sources of them in the diet, and provides recommendations for daily intake.

Chapter 2, "Fats": This chapter explains the functions of fats, covers the different types in the diet, and provides recommendations for daily intake.

Chapter 3, "Proteins": This chapter explains the functions of proteins and amino acids, covers the animal and plant sources in the diet, explains the effects of too little and too much dietary protein, and provides recommendations for daily intake.

Chapter 4, "Vitamins": This chapter provides an overview of the 13 vitamins and their functions and provides daily recommendations.

Chapter 5, "Minerals": This chapter provides an overview of the various types of vitamins in the diet and their functions and provides daily recommendations.

Chapter 6, "Creating a Daily Meal Plan": This chapter helps you determine your daily calorie needs and create an individualized meal plan based on the USDA's MyPyramid food guidance system.

Chapter 7, "Weight Management": This chapter provides an overview of energy balance, reviews the causes of and risks associated with being overweight or underweight, and provides dietary and physical activity tips to help you achieve and maintain a healthier body weight.

Chapter 8, "Eat to Beat Disease": This chapter reviews common diet-related diseases and conditions and provides dietary and lifestyle prevention strategies.

Chapter 9, "Food Allergies, Intolerances, and Sensitivities": This chapter explains common food allergies, food additive sensitivities, lactose intolerance, and gluten sensitivity and provides prevention and treatment strategies for each. It also provides a broad overview of food poisoning.

Chapter 10, "Healthy Food Shopping": This chapter helps you read and understand food labels and the various claims made on food packages, and provides an overview of functional foods, fat replacers, and sugar substitutes. It also includes an overview of dietary supplements.

Chapter 11, "Healthy Eating Tips": This chapter provides tips for increasing your fiber intake, and decreasing your intake of added sugar, saturated and trans fat, dietary cholesterol, and sodium.

Chapter 12, "Foodborne Illnesses and Food Safety": This chapter provides an overview of foodborne pathogens and other harmful substances in food. It also includes strategies to help you prevent foodborne illnesses as well as tips to help you safely shop, store, prepare, and cook food. In the back of this book, you'll find three appendixes:

▶ **Appendix A, "Words to Go Glossary":** This is a glossary of terms.

▶ **Appendix B, "Useful Resources":** This is a list of websites and organizations you can use or contact for more information.

▶ **Appendix C, "What's a Portion?":** This is a reference to help you estimate portion sizes for foods using common objects.

Acknowledgments

Thank you to Ruth Winter for recommending me for this project, Alison Fargis at The Stonesong Press for choosing me for this project, and my supportive literary agent Stacey Glick. To my wonderful sons, Spencer and Eli, who always encourage me to pursue the work I love and never make me feel guilty when I do. To Linda Arevalo for all she does to help me keep my home and life in order. To Andy Bellati and Sherina Wan for their wonderful research assistance for this project. To my one-of-a-kind parents Ron and Barbara Sickmen who are always first in line to brag of my accomplishments even though I repeatedly ask them not to. Finally, to my husband, Brian Zied: No words can express how I feel about him, an amazing person who never fails to love, encourage, and support me immensely, even when I get in my own way.

Special Thanks to the Technical Editor

Nutrition at Your Fingertips was reviewed by an expert who double-checked the accuracy of what you'll learn here, to help us ensure that this book gives you everything you need to know about nutrition. Special thanks are extended to the wonderful (and thorough) Susan Male Smith, M.A., R.D.

Trademarks

1

CARBOHYDRATES

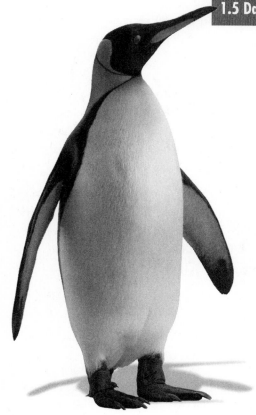

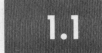 **FUNCTIONS OF CARBOHYDRATES**

In the Body
In the Diet

Carbohydrates are critical components of a healthy body and a well-balanced, nutritious diet. This subchapter covers the many important functions of carbohydrates in the body and in the diet.

In the Body

Carbohydrates provide the body with glucose, its key source of energy. The brain, red blood cells, and nervous system can use only glucose for fuel to perform their many functions. Most cells in the body use glucose to support breathing, contract and relax muscles (including the heart muscle), regulate body temperature and fluid balance, and support physical activity or exercise.

Provide Energy

As noted, the body breaks down carbohydrates into glucose, which provides energy. If your body makes more glucose than it needs for immediate energy, some is stored as **glycogen** either in your liver or in your muscles. Liver glycogen stores are used to regulate **blood glucose** (or **blood sugar**) levels, whereas muscle glycogen stores provide energy to fuel muscular work such as exercise.

Glycogen can be broken down and used for energy if you don't consume enough calories or sufficient dietary carbohydrates. Because no more than half a day's worth of glycogen can be stored in the body at any given time, it's important to regularly consume carbohydrate-rich foods and beverages to provide the energy you need for all your daily activities.

If your body makes more glucose than it needs for immediate energy or for storage, it is stored in your fat cells and becomes body fat.

Protect Body Proteins

If you consume too little carbohydrate, and at the same time you take in fewer calories than your body needs to maintain its weight, your body breaks down some of its proteins (including muscle tissue) to create glucose to fuel the brain, lungs, and many body cells. Losing muscle slows down your **metabolic rate** and makes it easier to gain weight (and harder to lose weight). Using body proteins

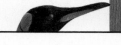
for energy doesn't let them perform some of their vital functions, including building and repairing muscle tissue, acting as enzymes or hormones, and supporting the immune system.

◀ *SEE ALSO 3.1, "Functions of Proteins"* ▶

◀ *SEE ALSO Chapter 7, "Weight Management"* ▶

To prevent your body from using proteins to create energy, you need to consume 50–100 grams of dietary carbohydrate each day. Here's what that looks like in terms of food:

▶ 50 grams of carbohydrate = 1 cup skim milk + ½ cup (16) grapes + 1 slice whole wheat bread + and ¼ cup kidney beans, cooked

▶ 100 grams of carbohydrate = 1½ cups strawberries + 1 cup whole wheat pasta + 1 cup low-fat yogurt + 2 tablespoons raisins + 1 small banana

Prevent Ketosis

Although carbohydrates supply the body with its main source of energy, fats can also play this role. However, the liver needs some dietary carbohydrate to fully break down fat into energy the body can use. When you don't consume enough dietary carbohydrate or have enough stored glycogen over a long period of time (for example, if you're starving, have cut your calories and/or carbohydrate intake too drastically, have diabetes, or have chronic alcoholism), your body creates small chemicals called **ketone bodies** that can be used for energy by most body cells. When your body makes more ketones than it needs for energy, a dangerous condition called **ketosis** can develop, increasing sodium and water loss from the body. This can cause symptoms such as nausea, weakness, and fatigue.

◀ *SEE ALSO 2.1, "Functions of Fats"* ▶

Help Regulate Blood Sugar Levels

Blood glucose (or blood sugar) levels are closely regulated to make sure your body cells have enough glucose for energy. If your blood sugar level is low, you can feel shaky or weak; if it's high, you can feel sluggish, confused, or short of breath. Blood sugar levels are tightly regulated by two hormones: insulin and glucagon.

After eating a meal, blood sugar levels rise. In response, the pancreas releases insulin into the blood. Insulin unlocks body cells, allowing the glucose to enter and provide them with energy. Insulin also stimulates cells in the liver and the muscles to store glucose in the form of glycogen for later use. During this process, blood sugar levels return to normal.

When you skip a meal or if you haven't eaten in a while, the pancreas releases another hormone, glucagon; glucagon stimulates the breakdown of glycogen from the liver into glucose, which is then released into the bloodstream. Glucagon also stimulates protein for glucose production.

In diabetes, the pancreas cannot release any or enough insulin into the bloodstream to bring blood sugar or blood glucose levels down to normal, and thus they are elevated.

◀ *SEE ALSO 8.3, "Diabetes"* ▶

In the Diet

Many foods and beverages that are widely available in the food supply and commonly consumed are rich in carbohydrates.

Dietary Sources

Carbohydrates are naturally found in a wide variety of plant foods and some animal-derived foods and beverages. These include

- ▶ Fruits
- ▶ Vegetables
- ▶ Grains
- ▶ Legumes (beans, including soybeans and foods and beverages made from soy, and peas)
- ▶ Milk and some milk products

◀ *SEE ALSO Chapter 6, "Creating a Daily Meal Plan"* ▶

Legumes (beans and peas), whole grains, fruits, and vegetables are great sources of fiber, which promotes gastrointestinal health and helps keep blood sugar and cholesterol levels in check.

◀ *SEE ALSO 1.4, "Dietary Fiber"* ▶

◀ *SEE ALSO 8.1, "Cardiovascular Disease"* ▶

These foods also supply the diet with an array of vitamins, minerals, and **phytochemicals** that can benefit health and protect against disease.

◀ *SEE ALSO Chapter 4, "Vitamins"* ▶

◀ *SEE ALSO Chapter 5, "Minerals"* ▶

Legumes (beans and peas), nuts, and seeds are also good sources of plant proteins. In particular, soybeans and foods made with them contain high-quality protein.

◀ *SEE ALSO 3.4, "Plant Sources of Protein"* ▶

Fruits, vegetables, and cooked grains are **nutrient-dense,** high in nutrients but low in calories. They add a lot of bulk for few calories because they have a high water content. Consequently, they can help you feel full with fewer calories.

◀ *SEE ALSO Chapter 7, "Weight Management"* ▶

Sugars and sugary foods are also significant sources of carbohydrates in the American diet. They can occur naturally (as in honey and even in milk and fruit) or be added to foods in refined forms (e.g., table sugar, molasses, and brown sugar). Foods rich in natural sugars, such as low fat or skim milk, and fruit (notably fresh, or frozen or canned with no added sugar), often pack in a lot of key nutrients. Oftentimes refined sugars are found in many of the nutrient-poor, high-calorie foods and beverages Americans tend to consume a lot of, including soda, cookies, and candy.

◀ *SEE ALSO 1.2, "Sugars"* ▶

Different carbohydrate-rich foods have different effects on blood sugar levels. Foods that are rich in simple carbohydrates or starch and are low in fiber and fat are more rapidly digested and absorbed; this leads to a large, rapid rise in blood sugar levels. The body responds by pumping out extra insulin that can lower blood sugar levels too far before finally stabilizing.

Carbohydrate-rich foods that are high in fiber, resistant starch, and fat cause a less dramatic rise and fall in blood sugar.

◀ *SEE ALSO 1.3, "Starch"* ▶

Glycogen is the storage form of glucose, a simple sugar and the body's main source of energy or fuel.

Blood glucose or **blood sugar** is the amount of glucose (a simple sugar found in foods and also made and stored in the body) that's found in the blood. Glucose is the body's main source of energy and the brain's only source.

Metabolic rate is the rate at which the body converts food into energy it can use.

Ketone bodies are toxic chemicals made by the body when fat is used instead of sugar to create glucose, the body's main source of energy.

Ketosis is a condition that results from the incomplete breakdown of body fat to be used for energy. During ketosis, ketone bodies accumulate in the bloodstream and body tissues.

Phytochemicals are compounds in plants that are not essential to life, but that have healthful effects. These compounds may also affect the taste, color, and smell of foods.

Nutrient-dense foods are those that contain a lot of nutrients for relatively few calories.

1.2 SUGARS

Overview

Two Types

Nutritive Sweeteners

Refined Sugars

Sugar Alcohols

In this subchapter, you are introduced to the two types of simple sugars found in the diet. You also learn about the naturally occurring and refined sugars as well as sugar alcohols found in, or added to, foods and beverages.

Overview

A variety of foods and beverages contain simple sugars. Some are naturally occurring, but many are created through refining and added to processed foods and beverages to enhance their taste, smell, texture, and color. Whatever their source, all sugars are treated the same way by the body; they're all broken down into glucose to provide energy. All sugars provide 4 calories per gram.

Two Types

The two main categories of simple sugars in foods are monosaccharides and disaccharides.

Monosaccharides

Monosaccharides are simple carbohydrates that contain one single unit of sugar. The three common monosaccharides found in the diet are glucose, fructose, and galactose.

Glucose, also called dextrose, adds a mildly sweet taste to foods. In foods, it is often found paired with another monosaccharide to form a disaccharide or a double sugar unit; for example, glucose and galactose are linked together to form lactose, the main sugar found in milk and milk products.

◁ SEE ALSO 6.7, *"Milk"* ▷

In the body, glucose provides the brain, nervous system, and many body cells with their main source of energy.

◁ SEE ALSO 1.1, *"Functions of Carbohydrates"* ▷

7

Fructose, also known as fruit sugar or levulose, is the sweetest sugar. Fructose is found in fruits, some vegetables, table sugar, and honey. Fructose and glucose are also found in high-fructose corn syrup, a caloric sweetener used in a variety of commonly consumed foods and beverages.

Some people are unable to digest fructose because of fructose intolerance, a rare genetic disorder; many others can have **fructose malabsorption** and experience bloating, abdominal pain, diarrhea, and other gastrointestinal symptoms.

◀ *SEE ALSO Chapter 9, "Food Allergies, Intolerances, and Sensitivities"* ▶

Galactose, another monosaccharide, is rarely found in foods by itself but is attached to glucose to create lactose, the main sugar found in milk and milk products.

Disaccharides

Disaccharides are made of two monosaccharides (single units of sugar) linked together. The disaccharides found in foods and beverages are sucrose, lactose, and maltose.

Sucrose, also known as table sugar, is made when glucose is paired with fructose. It is extracted from sugar beet or sugar cane plants and is purified and refined to create white table sugar. Molasses is also created from the sugar-refining process; brown sugar is white sugar turned brown through the addition of molasses. Sucrose is also added to a variety of foods and beverages, including soda; baked goods such as cookies, cakes, and pies; ready-to-eat cereals; dairy foods; canned fruit; and others.

Lactose, commonly known as milk sugar, is made up of glucose and galactose. It is naturally found in milk, cheese, and yogurt, and in foods and beverages made with them. Lactose is added as an ingredient to a variety of processed foods, beverages, and even medications.

People with lactose intolerance are unable to digest small amounts of lactose. This occurs because their bodies don't make enough of the enzyme lactase, which breaks down lactose into its simple sugars: glucose and galactose. People with lactose intolerance can experience cramps, nausea, bloating, gas, or other symptoms when they consume milk, cheese, yogurt, or any lactose-containing foods or beverages.

◀ *SEE ALSO 9.3, "Lactose Intolerance"* ▶

Maltose, also known as malt or malt sugar, is made of two glucose units joined together. It is created when starches, long chains of monosaccharides, are broken down in the body into two glucose units. Maltose is found in some commercial cereals and baked goods and is fermented to make beer.

◀ *SEE ALSO 1.3, "Starch"* ▶

Nutritive Sweeteners

Unlike artificial sweeteners that have few or no calories, nutritive sweeteners contain calories. Simple sugars (monosaccharides and disaccharides) and **sugar alcohols** can come from natural or refined sources; high-fructose corn syrup, another nutritive sweetener, is commercially created and used in a variety of foods and beverages.

◀ *SEE ALSO 10.4, "Fat Replacers and Sugar Substitutes"* ▶

Naturally Occurring Sugars

Here are some examples of naturally occurring sugars in foods and beverages:

- ▶ Fructose (in fruit)
- ▶ Lactose (in milk and milk products)
- ▶ Fructose plus glucose (in honey)
- ▶ Sucrose (in real maple syrup)

As you can see, some foods and beverages that contain naturally occurring sugars also deliver many nutrients and other healthful substances. For example, fruit is a rich source of fiber, vitamins, minerals, and phytochemicals; milk and milk products, especially low-fat and nonfat varieties, provide calcium, vitamin D, and high-quality protein.

◀ *SEE ALSO 6.3, "Fruit"* ▶

◀ *SEE ALSO 6.7, "Milk"* ▶

Refined Sugars

Some nutritive sweeteners are not found naturally but instead are created commercially. During refining, monosaccharides and disaccharides are extracted from plant foods to create sugars that can be added to foods, such as white table sugar, molasses, brown sugar, and high-fructose corn syrup.

These sugars provide calories but few nutrients; they are often added to, or found in, foods and beverages that are high in calories but low in key nutrients. It's important to keep your intake of **added sugars** low to leave room for more healthful foods and beverages.

◀ SEE ALSO 1.5, "Daily Carbohydrate Recommendations" ▶

High-fructose corn syrup (HFCS) is the main calorie-containing sweetener used in America. Although the biggest dietary source is nondiet soda, HFCS is also found in many foods and beverages including salad dressings, pickled products, ketchup, baked foods such as breads, tabletop syrups, candies, gums, desserts, and fruit drinks.

In recent years, HFCS has been singled out as a possible contributor to the current obesity epidemic in America. Some argue that increased availability of HFCS in our food supply has contributed significantly to an increased intake of sugar. Surveys have shown that obesity rates have climbed in both adults and children, in part due to increased daily calorie intake, and many of those calories come from sugary soda and other foods and beverages made with added sugars including HFCS.

Although some researchers believe that, compared with equal calorie amounts of other sugars and sweeteners, consuming fructose (in the form of HFCS) affects hormones in a way that increases appetite and promotes body fat accumulation, recent research has failed to confirm this.

A recent report by The American Medical Association (AMA) concluded it's unlikely that HFCS contributes more to obesity or other conditions than sucrose. Still, the AMA, the United States Department of Agriculture's Dietary Guidelines for Americans and **MyPyramid,** and many health professionals urge Americans to significantly reduce their intake of added sugars from all sources to stay within recommended guidelines.

◀ SEE ALSO 6.2, "Your Daily Meal Pattern" ▶

◀ SEE ALSO 6.9, "Discretionary Calories" ▶

Because HFCS is found in a lot of high-calorie, nutrient-poor foods and beverages, and because foods with added sugars tend to be easy to overconsume, reducing your intake of any foods high in HFCS or any added sugars and sweeteners can certainly help reduce your overall calorie intake and leave room for more healthful foods and beverages.

Sugar Alcohols

Sugar alcohols, also known as polyols, are found naturally in a variety of fruits and vegetables. They're also commercially made from sucrose and glucose (two simple sugars) and from starch (a polysaccharide).

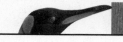

Sugar alcohols add sweetness, bulk, texture, and moisture to foods and are often used by manufacturers to create reduced or low-carbohydrate products that appeal to people with type 2 diabetes or who simply want to limit their dietary carbohydrate intake. In general, sugar alcohols differ from sugar in that they're not as sweet (though sweetness varies), have less of an impact on blood sugar levels than simple sugars, are less likely to promote tooth decay, and provide only about half as many calories (about 2 calories per gram versus 4 in sucrose and other sugars) because they're only partially digested and absorbed by the body. (Erythritol is unique in that it is virtually calorie-free.)

Some examples of sugar alcohols commonly found in foods and beverages include erythritol, lactilol, mannitol, sorbitol, and xylitol.

Because sugar alcohols are incompletely digested and therefore fermented by bacteria, consuming too many products that contain them can cause diarrhea, bloating, and abdominal pain because they're in the large intestine. Again, erythritol is an exception; it's less likely to cause diarrhea than other polyols.

WORDS TO GO . . . WORDS TO GO . . . WORDS TO GO

Fructose malabsorption is a condition in which fructose cannot be absorbed into the bloodstream and instead stays in the gastrointestinal tract unabsorbed; this can cause gastrointestinal symptoms such as bloating, diarrhea, and abdominal pain.

Sugar alcohols are compounds that contain monosaccharides (simple sugars) and are often used as nutritive sweeteners in many processed foods.

Added sugars are sugars and syrups added to foods during processing or when preparing, cooking, or consuming foods at the table.

MyPyramid is a graphic representation of the Dietary Guidelines for Americans, a set of science-based recommendations for how to eat well to promote health and prevent disease. MyPyramid replaced the previous Food Guide Pyramid; it recommends specific calorie levels and meal patterns using foods and beverages from several categories.

1.3 STARCH

In the Body

In the Diet

Modified Starch

In this subchapter, you learn about the types of starch, complex carbohydrates found in the body and diet. You also learn which foods are good sources of starch.

In the Body

Some of the starch derived from complex carbohydrate-rich foods in the diet is stored in the human body.

Glycogen

Glycogen, also known as animal starch, is the term given to stored glucose in the body reserved for future use as energy. When your body makes or has more glucose than it needs for immediate energy, some of it is converted to glycogen and stored in two places: in the liver and in the muscles.

The glycogen stored in the liver can be used to keep blood glucose or blood sugar levels steady, and the glycogen stored in muscle tissue can be used as an energy source during strenuous exercise or physical activity.

Because your body can't store unlimited amounts of glycogen—only about 200–500 grams of glycogen, or up to half a day's worth—it's critical to consume a variety of carbohydrate-rich foods throughout the day and enough total calories to meet your daily glucose needs.

◄ SEE ALSO 1.1, *"Functions of Carbohydrates"* ►

◄ SEE ALSO 6.2, *"Your Daily Meal Pattern"* ►

In the Diet

Starch is made up of many units of glucose strung together to form a polysaccharide (a complex carbohydrate). Like sugars, most starches are digested, absorbed, and used for short-term energy or stored. Starch is found naturally in plants. Glucose is stored in the starch and used to help plants grow well and reproduce.

Sources

Starch is naturally found in plant foods including grains (such as wheat, rice, corn, oats, millet, and barley), legumes (beans, peas, lentils, lima beans, black-eyed peas, and pinto beans), and tubers (potatoes, yams, and cassava).

◀ SEE ALSO 3.4, *"Plant Sources of Protein"* ▶

◀ SEE ALSO 6.4, *"Vegetables"* ▶

◀ SEE ALSO 6.5, *"Grains"* ▶

◀ SEE ALSO 6.6, *"Meat and Beans"* ▶

Starch is found in foods in two main forms: amylopectin and amylose.

In most starchy foods, about 70–80 percent of the starch comes from **amylopectin** and the remaining 20–30 percent from **amylose.** In some foods, such as barley, corn, and rice, the ratio of amylopectin to amylose can vary. And some foods, like waxy barley and rice, contain almost all amylopectin, while some foods like wheat flour have more amylose than amylopectin. Of both types of starch, amylose is thought to be less digestible than amylopectin.

Although the body can easily digest most starches, some remain trapped in plant cells and cannot be digested in the small intestine. These starches, known as **resistant starches,** fall into the category of fiber and can have similar health benefits. Although some resistant starches are naturally found in foods, manufacturers are increasingly making resistant starches from corn, wheat, and potatoes and adding as a form of fiber to a variety of foods including breads, cereals, pasta, crackers, and other carbohydrate-rich foods.

◀ SEE ALSO 1.4, *"Dietary Fiber"* ▶

Modified Starch

Modified starch is a food additive created by degrading starch using several methods. It's commonly used to moisten, thicken, stabilize, or emulsify foods including frozen products, salad dressings, batter, and jellybeans (forms the outer shell). Modified starches are also sometimes found in medications.

Amylopectin is one of two main components of starch (the other is amylose); it is made up of branched chains of polysaccharides (long chains that contain more than 10 glucose units).

Amylose is one of two main components of starch (the other is amylopectin); it is made up of straight chains of polysaccharides (long chains that contain more than 10 glucose units).

Resistant starches are a type of fiber; they include starches and products of the breakdown of starch that are not absorbed in the small intestines of healthy individuals.

1.4 DIETARY FIBER

Definition

Sources

Health Benefits

Health Risks

Fiber is found naturally in all plant foods and is increasingly added to processed foods to provide some health benefits. In this subchapter, you learn what fiber is and which foods are good sources of it. You also learn about the many health benefits fiber has to offer and the potential problems of consuming too much of it.

Definition

Fiber is classified as complex carbohydrates (more than two sugar units linked together).

In 2002, the Institute of Medicine created the following definitions for fiber, separating it into three components: dietary fiber, functional fiber, and total fiber:

▶ Dietary fiber—Includes carbohydrates and lignins (the noncarbohydrate components of vegetables, such as the woody components of carrots or the seeds found in strawberries) found naturally in plants that our bodies cannot digest or absorb.

▶ Functional fiber—Includes isolated, manufactured, or synthetic oligosaccharides (complex carbohydrates that contain 3–10 sugar or glucose units) that our bodies cannot digest or absorb and that have beneficial health effects (for example, it can improve regularity, improve blood sugar and dietary cholesterol levels, and reduce disease risk).

▶ Total fiber—Is the sum of dietary fiber and functional fiber.

Nutrition Facts Labels on food packages currently list dietary fiber under total carbohydrates and further distinguish dietary fiber as **soluble** or **insoluble fiber.** According to the Institute of Medicine, the scientific support for using solubility to determine beneficial health effects is inconsistent, and recent studies suggest that other characteristics of fiber—including fermentability and viscosity—can be important to consider. Because of this, the Institute of Medicine recommends that the terms *soluble* and *insoluble* no longer be used.

◀ SEE ALSO 10.1, *"Reading Food Labels"* ▶

Sources

Fiber is found in a variety of plant foods. Legumes (beans and peas), grains (especially whole grains), fruits, and vegetables all contribute fiber to the diet. Following are some top food sources of fiber; choosing many of these each day can help you meet your daily recommended intake for fiber of 25 grams.

TOP FOOD SOURCES OF FIBER

Food	Amount	Fiber (g)
Barley, pearled, raw	1 cup	31
Bulgur, dry	1 cup	26
Beans, navy, cooked	1 cup	19
Peas, split, cooked	1 cup	16
Lentils, mature seeds, cooked	1 cup	16
Wheat flour, whole-grain	1 cup	15
Oat bran, raw	1 cup	15
Artichokes (globe or French), cooked	1 cup	14
Beans, kidney, red, canned	1 cup	14
Chickpeas, cooked	1 cup	13
Buckwheat flour	1 cup	12
Soybeans, mature, cooked	1 cup	10
Pears, Asian, raw	1 pear	10
Cornmeal, self-rising, enriched, yellow	1 cup	10
Couscous, dry	1 cup	9
Vegetables, mixed, frozen, cooked	1 cup	8
Raspberries, raw	1 cup	8
Blackberries, raw	1 cup	8
Nuts, chestnuts, roasted	1 cup	7
Spinach, frozen, cooked	1 cup	7
Lettuce, iceberg	1 head	7
Brussels sprouts, frozen, cooked	1 cup	6
Barley, pearled, cooked	1 cup	6
Squash, winter, all varieties, baked	1 cup	6
Parsnips, boiled	1 cup	6
Turnip greens, frozen, cooked	1 cup	6
Broccoli, frozen, cooked	1 cup	6
Papayas, raw	1	6

Food	Amount	Fiber (g)
Collards, cooked	1 cup	5
Okra, frozen, cooked	1 cup	5
Broccoli, cooked	1 cup	5
Cauliflower, frozen, cooked	1 cup	5
Carrots, cooked	1 cup	5
Potato, baked, flesh and skin	1 (7 oz.)	4
Spinach, cooked	1 cup	4
Oranges, all varieties	1 cup	4
Beet greens, cooked	1 cup	4
Beans, snap, yellow, cooked	1 cup	4
Plantains, raw	1 (6 oz.)	4
Rice, white, long-grain	1 cup	4
Rice, brown, long-grain, cooked	1 cup	4
Blueberries, raw	1 cup	4
Nuts, almonds	24	4
Mushrooms, cooked	1 cup	3
Figs, dried, uncooked	2	3
Apples, raw, with skin	1	3
Peppers, sweet, red, raw	1 cup	3
Carrots, raw	1 cup	3

Source: U.S. Department of Agriculture, Agricultural Research Service. 2008. USDA National Nutrient Database for Standard Reference, Release 21. Nutrient Data Laboratory Home Page at www.ars.usda. gov/ba/bhnrc/ndl.

◄ SEE ALSO 1.5, "Daily Carbohydrate Recommendations" ►

Resistant Starch

Resistant starch is a type of dietary fiber. Resistant starch is defined as the sum of starch and products of starch degradation (breakdown of starch) that's not absorbed in the small intestine of a healthy individual.

Resistant starch is found naturally in a variety of plant foods or it is added to processed foods. The four main dietary sources of resistant starch include

- ► Whole-grain foods (whole or partly milled grains and seeds)
- ► Raw potatoes, unripe bananas, some legumes, and in high-amylose starches such as those obtained from high-amylose corn

▶ Cooked and cooled foods, such as potatoes, bread, and cornflakes

▶ Processed foods made with resistant starches

◀ *SEE ALSO 1.3, "Starch"* ▶

The amount of resistant starch in foods varies widely; our estimated daily intake ranges from about 3 grams to about 8 grams per day. Studies suggest that consuming 6–12 grams of resistant starch at a meal can benefit glucose and insulin levels after the meal; consuming 20 grams per day has also been shown to bulk up feces and benefit digestive health.

Fiber Supplements

Fiber supplements are often sold as bran tablets or purified **cellulose** or in the form of laxatives (stool softeners). Whether in pill, powder, or drink form, fiber supplements can help some people consume adequate amounts of fiber. But taking fiber supplements (or eating fiber-fortified foods) makes overconsuming fiber easy, and too much can cause gastrointestinal symptoms. Fiber supplements do not replace a diet rich in plant foods that naturally contain fiber along with other key nutrients and substances that benefit health.

◀ *SEE ALSO 10.5, "Dietary Supplements"* ▶

Health Benefits

Studies have shown that people who consume more dietary fiber also tend to weigh less. That's no surprise because many high-fiber foods, especially those that contain a lot of water such as fruits, vegetables, and cooked grains, are very filling. Eating a lot of fiber-rich foods such as legumes; whole grains; and other fiber-rich grains, fruits, and vegetables can help you lower your total daily calorie intake.

◀ *SEE ALSO Chapter 6, "Creating a Daily Meal Plan"* ▶

Consuming a fiber-rich diet can also help you steady your blood sugar levels and keep you energized throughout the day. It can also help you manage, lower your risk of, or treat obesity, cardiovascular disease, and cancer as well as gastrointestinal conditions such as constipation.

◀ *SEE ALSO Chapter 8, "Eat to Beat Disease"* ▶

Health Risks

Too much dietary fiber can reduce the absorption of vitamins, minerals, proteins, and energy. It can also cause symptoms such as abdominal pain, flatulence, bloating, and diarrhea if consumed in excessive amounts. To minimize these symptoms, as people incorporate more fiber into their diet to meet current recommendations, they should also take in more water and other fluids to ease the passage of fiber throughout the body.

◀ SEE ALSO 1.5, *"Daily Carbohydrate Recommendations"* ▶

◀ SEE ALSO 6.10, *"Daily Water Needs"* ▶

WORDS TO GO . . .WORDS TO GO . . .WORDS TO GO

Soluble fiber is not digested by the human body; it absorbs and retains water and forms a gel-like substance.

Insoluble fiber is not digested by the human body; it does not absorb and retain water like soluble fiber but stays intact as it passes through the body.

Cellulose is a straight-chain polysaccharide (more than two units of glucose joined together); it is the main component of plant cell walls and is not digested in the human body.

1.5 DAILY CARBOHYDRATE RECOMMENDATIONS

Total Digestible Carbohydrates
Total Fiber

In this subchapter, you learn how to calculate your individual daily carbohydrate and fiber needs.

Total Digestible Carbohydrates

According to the **Dietary Reference Intakes (DRI)**, digestible carbohydrates (including starches and both naturally occurring and added sugars) should make up about 45–65 percent of total daily calorie intake for Americans age 1 and over. This recommendation reflects the **Acceptable Macronutrient Distribution Range (AMDR)**, the recommended range of daily carbohydrate intake.

Here's how you can figure out how many calories should come from total digestible carbohydrates:

1. Multiply your daily calorie intake by 0.45 (45%) to determine the lower end of the calorie range.

2. Multiply your daily calorie intake by 0.65 (65%).

For example, if you need 1,600 calories per day to maintain a healthy body weight or to promote weight loss, here's how you'd figure out how many calories from carbohydrate-rich foods to aim for:

1. 1,600 multiplied by 0.45 equals 720 calories.

2. 1,600 multiplied by 0.65 equals 1,040 calories.

Based on these calculations, your daily calorie range for total digestible carbohydrate intake should be between 720 and 1,040 calories. To determine how many grams of carbohydrates that equals, do the following:

Divide both numbers by 4 calories (because there are 4 calories per gram of carbohydrate).

720 calories divided by 4 calories equals 180 grams of carbohydrate.

1,040 calories divided by 4 calories equals 260 grams of carbohydrate.

So your daily goal should be 180–260 grams of total digestible carbohydrates.

Here is an approximation for the number of grams of carbohydrate in a portion according to the MyPyramid Food Guidance System based on the Dietary Guidelines for Americans:

▶ Grains—A 1-ounce equivalent has approximately 15 grams of carbohydrate.

▶ Fruit—½ cup has approximately 15 grams of carbohydrate.

▶ Milk or yogurt—A 1-cup equivalent has about 12 grams of carbohydrate.

▶ Vegetable—½ cup has about 5 grams of carbohydrate.

◁ *SEE ALSO 6.2, "Your Daily Meal Pattern"* ▷

The following are the daily total digestible carbohydrate intake recommendations for American children and adults. The goals for infants are based on **adequate intakes (AI)**, and those for children and adults are based on **recommended dietary allowances (RDA)**:

RECOMMENDED DAILY INTAKE
FOR TOTAL DIGESTIBLE CARBOHYDRATES

Age	Amount (g)	Age	Amount (g)
Infants		**Women**	
0–6 months	60	Not pregnant or	
7–12 months	95	lactating, 19–70+ years	130
Children		Pregnant	175
1–18 years	130	Lactating	210
Men			
19–70+ years	130		

Source: Dietary Reference Intakes for Energy, Carbohydrate, Fiber, Fat, Fatty Acids, Cholesterol, Protein, and Amino Acids (2002).

Following the MyPyramid daily meal pattern will help you meet and not exceed the recommendations for total digestible carbohydrates.

Added sugars are part of the 45–65 percent range for total digestible carbohydrate intake. According to MyPyramid, added sugars count as discretionary calories. You can consume all or part of your total discretionary calorie allotment (which ranges from 165 to 648 calories depending on your daily recommended total calorie intake) from added sugars as long as all your other daily food choices are in their lowest fat and lowest sugar forms.

◄ SEE ALSO 6.1, *"Estimating Your Daily Calorie Needs"* ►

◄ SEE ALSO 6.2, *"Your Daily Meal Plan"* ►

◄ SEE ALSO 6.9, *"Discretionary Calories"* ►

Total Fiber

The Institute of Medicine (IOM) set the following AI recommendation for daily fiber intake:

14 grams per 1000 calories

This AI is based on evidence that this level can decrease the risk of chronic diseases and other health-related conditions.

◄ SEE ALSO 8.1, *"Cardiovascular Disease"* ►

Here are more specific fiber recommendations for infants, children, and adults based on AI. These fiber recommendations reflect daily amounts shown to reduce the risk of coronary heart disease:

DAILY INTAKE OF FIBER

Age and Stage	Amount (g)	Age and Stage	Amount (g)
Infants		**Females**	
0–6 months	ND*	9–13 years	26
7–12 months	ND*	14–18 years	26
Children		19–30 years	25
1–3 years	19	31–50 years	25
4–8 years	25	51–70 years	21
Males		Older than 70 years	21
9–13 years	31	**Pregnancy**	
14–18 years	38	18 years or younger	28
19–30 years	38	19–30 years	28
31–50 years	38	31–50 years	28
51–70 years	30	**Lactation**	
70 years	30	18 years or younger	29
		19–30 years	29
		31–50 years	29

*ND = not determinable due to lack of data of adverse effects in this age group and with regard to lack of ability to handle excess amounts. Source of intake should be from food only to prevent high levels of intake.

Source: Dietary Reference Intakes from Energy, Carbohydrates, Fiber, Fat, Fatty Acids, Cholesterol, Protein, and Amino Acids (2002/2005). www.nap.edu.

Dietary reference intakes (DRIs) is a set of four reference values for essential vitamins and minerals based on observational and clinical studies; it includes the estimated average requirements (EARs), recommended dietary allowances (RDAs), adequate intakes (AIs), and tolerable upper intake levels (ULs).

Acceptable macronutrient distribution range (AMDR) is the range of intake for a particular calorie-containing nutrient (carbohydrate, fat, or protein) that provides enough of that essential nutrient while reducing the risk of chronic disease; if an individual exceeds the AMDR for any nutrient, the risk of chronic disease and/or insufficient nutrient intake increases.

Adequate intake (AI) is an estimate of the needs of a particular nutrient for most healthy people; it is used when there is not enough scientific data to create RDAs for that nutrient.

Recommended dietary allowance (RDA) is the average daily amount of a nutrient that is sufficient to meet the requirement for nearly all healthy people at each stage of life.

2
FATS

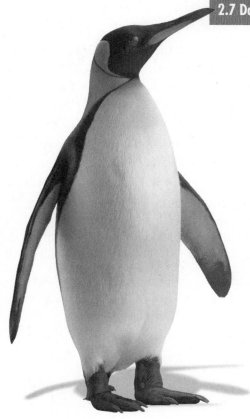

2.1 FUNCTIONS OF FATS

In the Body
In the Diet

In this subchapter, you learn the many key roles fat plays in both the body and the diet.

In the Body

Fats provide the body with a key source of energy. Although glucose is the main source of energy for the brain and nervous system, muscle tissues prefer fats for energy. During exercise, muscles rely on fats for energy after glucose and glycogen (stored glucose) have been depleted.

◄ SEE ALSO 1.1, *"Functions of Carbohydrates"* ▷

Fats also insulate and protect our bodies and vital organs, including the brain. About 15–30 percent of our total body weight comes from stored fat. The two main types of fat in our bodies are visceral fat and subcutaneous fat.

Visceral fat is buried below the body's muscle tissue. It surrounds vital organs to cushion and protect them. Women usually have more body visceral fat than men and tend to store more in their breasts, hips, and thighs as a way of protecting organs involved in reproduction. Having excess visceral fat in the lower part of the body appears to be less harmful than having it in the abdominal area, where men tend to accumulate it. Visceral fat in the abdominal area is believed to secrete powerful chemicals that can increase the risk for diseases such as heart disease, diabetes, hypertension, metabolic syndrome, and breathing problems.

◄ SEE ALSO Chapter 8, *"Eat to Beat Disease"* ▷

Subcutaneous fat is the fat you can see; it lies just beneath the skin. This fat also protects and insulates the body.

Fats also carry some important vitamins (including vitamins A, D, E, and K), **carotenoids,** and other substances that dissolve in fat to help them be better absorbed and used by the body.

◄ SEE ALSO 4.2, *"Vitamin A"* ▷

◄ SEE ALSO 4.3, *"Vitamin D"* ▷

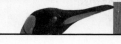

◄ *SEE ALSO 4.4, "Vitamin E"* ▶

◄ *SEE ALSO 4.5, "Vitamin K"* ▶

Fats are also used to create and maintain cell membranes (the outer layer or cells that protect them) and help maintain healthy skin and nails.

2.1

In the Diet

Dietary fats, also known as dietary **triglycerides,** are found in a variety of foods from both animal and plant sources. They are more than twice as energy-dense as the other macronutrients: carbohydrate and protein. Fat provides 9 calories per gram, although carbohydrate and protein each contain only 4 calories per gram. (Incidentally, alcohol, not a nutrient but still a source of calories, falls somewhere in between and provides 7 calories per gram.)

Fats also promote *satiety,* or the feeling of fullness. Fats in foods add a lot to their taste, texture, smell, and mouth feel. Fats in foods are versatile, can be heated to high temperatures without degrading, and can be used in countless cooking methods to create highly palatable foods.

If you consume too much dietary fat, your body can efficiently store it as body fat. This stored fat can be easily accessed when your calorie needs increase—for example, during periods of growth (such as in pregnancy or childhood), during illness or after an injury, or during a natural disaster or at times when food is scarce. In normal circumstances, too much dietary fat can put you at risk for being overweight or for obesity, and too much of certain types of fats (including saturated and trans fats) can contribute to the development of heart disease and other diet-related diseases and conditions.

◄ *SEE ALSO 2.4, "Saturated Fats"* ▶

◄ *SEE ALSO 2.5, "Trans Fats"* ▶

◄ *SEE ALSO Chapter 7, "Weight Management"* ▶

◄ *SEE ALSO Chapter 8, "Eat to Beat Disease"* ▶

If you consume too little dietary fat, your body fat stores can become depleted. If you're a woman, you might stop menstruating and have reproductive problems. Your skin might deteriorate, you might feel cold (because you have less body fat to warm you), and your organs and tissues might be at more risk for injury. This can be a problem, especially for older people who might have a chronic disease. Children who don't consume enough fat (it's rare, but can happen) won't get enough essential fats that they need to get from the diet. If they don't consume enough calories, they don't accumulate/have enough body fat (everybody needs some body fat!), and they can literally stop growing. A deficiency is rare especially in the United States, but still kids need enough fat to grow optimally.

WORDS TO GO . . .WORDS TO GO . . .WORDS TO GO

Carotenoids are a group of yellow, orange, and red pigments found in plant foods (most often in fruits and vegetables). They act as antioxidants to protect body cells against damage caused by free radicals (harmful substances found in the body and environment).

Triglycerides are made of three fatty acids joined to a glycerol unit (an alcohol that forms the backbone of triglycerides). Triglycerides are found in fats and oils and foods made with them as well as in meats, dairy products, nuts, and seeds.

2.2   MONOUNSATURATED FATS

Definition and Dietary Sources

Health Implications

In this subchapter, you learn what monounsaturated fats are and the types found in foods. You also learn why these fats are healthful dietary components.

Definition and Dietary Sources

Monounsaturated fats, like all dietary fats, provide the body with an efficient energy source. These fats are in liquid form at room temperature but can become more solid when refrigerated. The two types of monounsaturated fats found in the diet are oleic acid and palmitoleic acid.

Oleic acid is the main source of monounsaturated fats found in foods. Key food sources for these fats include

- ▶ Vegetable oils (olive oil, canola oil, peanut oil, mid-oleic sunflower oil, and other mid- and high-oleic vegetable oils)
- ▶ Nuts and seeds (including almonds, cashews, pistachios, and peanuts)
- ▶ Olives
- ▶ Avocados

Palmitoleic acid is found in macadamia nuts, some fish oils, and beef fat.

Here's how much total monounsaturated fat you'll find in some commonly consumed foods:

FOOD SOURCES OF MONOUNSATURATED FATS (MUFAS)

Food	Amount	MUFAs (g)
Nuts, macadamia, dry-roasted	10–12	17
Avocado, sliced	½ cup	14
Nuts, hazelnuts or filberts	28	13
Nuts, pecans	20 halves	12
Oil, vegetable, safflower, high-oleic	1 tbsp.	10
Oil, olive	1 tbsp.	10
Avocado	½	10
Nuts, mixed, with peanuts, dry-roasted	1 oz.	9

continues

29

FOOD SOURCES OF MONOUNSATURATED FATS
(MUFAS) (CONTINUED)

Food	Amount	MUFAs (g)
Oil, vegetable, canola	1 tbsp.	9
Nuts, almonds	24	9
Nuts, cashews, dry-roasted	1 oz.	8
Peanuts, dry-roasted	28	7
Nuts, Brazil nuts, dried	6–8	7
Nuts, pistachio nuts, dry-roasted	47	7
Oil, peanut	1 tbsp.	6
Oil, soybean	1 tbsp.	6
Oil, sesame	1 tbsp.	5
Nuts, pine nuts, dried	1 oz.	5

Source: U.S. Department of Agriculture, Agricultural Research Service. 2008. USDA National Nutrient Database for Standard Reference, Release 21. Nutrient Data Laboratory Home Page, www.ars.usda.gov/ba/bhnrc/ndl.

Health Implications

Many foods that are rich in monounsaturated fats are also good or excellent sources of other key nutrients (for example, vegetable oils are rich sources of vitamin E, and nuts and seeds provide plant protein, fiber, and some vitamins and minerals).

� SEE ALSO 3.4, *"Plant Sources of Protein"* ▶

� SEE ALSO 4.4, *"Vitamin E"* ▶

Studies have shown that replacing saturated fats with monounsaturated and polyunsaturated fats (although keeping calories consistent) can lower bad low-density lipoprotein (LDL) **cholesterol** levels. This can protect cholesterol from accumulating in the linings of arteries that lead to the heart or the brain and can cause a heart attack or stroke, respectively.

� SEE ALSO 2.3, *"Polyunsaturated Fats"* ▶

� SEE ALSO 8.1, *"Cardiovascular Disease"* ▶

A recent review of several studies found that those who consumed a high-fat diet with 22–33 percent energy from monounsaturated fats lowered their total blood cholesterol, very low-density lipoprotein cholesterol, and blood triglycerides more than those who consumed a low-fat, high-carbohydrate diet.

Too much of any fat—even healthful monounsaturated fat—can lead to excess calorie intake and contribute to the development of being overweight or obesity. That can increase the risk of diet-related diseases including heart disease, high blood pressure, and type 2 diabetes.

◄ *SEE ALSO 2.7, "Daily Fat and Cholesterol Recommendations"* ►

◄ *SEE ALSO Chapter 7, "Weight Management"* ►

◄ *SEE ALSO Chapter 8, "Eat to Beat Disease"* ►

2.2

WORDS TO GO . . .WORDS TO GO . . .WORDS TO GO

Cholesterol is a fatlike substance that is present in all animal tissues.

2.3 POLYUNSATURATED FATS

Definition and Dietary Sources
Health Implications

In this subchapter, you learn what polyunsaturated fats are and which foods are rich sources. You also learn the health benefits and potential risks associated with the intake of polyunsaturated fats.

Definitions and Dietary Sources

Polyunsaturated fats are essential fats the body can't make and needs to obtain from the diet. They are usually in liquid form at room temperature or when refrigerated.

The two main categories of polyunsaturated fats found in foods are omega-6 fats and omega-3 fats.

Omega-6 fats provide readily available energy to the body as well as essential fats the body needs but cannot create. Three main types of omega-6 fats are found in foods: linoleic acid (LA), arachidonic acid (AA), and conjugated linoleic acid (CLA).

Linoleic acid is the key source of polyunsaturated fats in the diet and is found in the food supply in sunflower, safflower, corn, cottonseed, and soybean oils. Arachidonic acid is found in small amounts in meats, poultry, and egg yolk, and conjugated linoleic acid is found in butterfat and meat.

Omega-3 fats also provide our bodies with energy and essential fats. They're also linked with heart health and other benefits.

Three different types of omega-3 fats are found in foods: eicosapentaenoic acid (EPA) and docosapaentanoic acid (DHA) are long-chain omega-3 fats found in fish, and alpha-linolenic acid (ALA) is a short-chain fatty acid found in plant foods. Here are some common food sources of each:

▶ EPA and DHA: Cold-water fatty fish such as salmon, tuna, trout, mackerel, herring, and oysters

▶ ALA: Soybean oil, canola oil, flaxseed oil, flaxseeds, walnuts, and tofu

In the body, very small amounts of ALA can be converted to EPA and DHA.

Several foods and beverages, including ready-to-eat cereals and dairy foods, are also fortified with EPA, DHA, and/or ALA, although the amounts contained in such products are often small.

◀ *SEE ALSO 10.3, "Functional Foods"* ▶

Health Implications

Foods rich in polyunsaturated fats provide energy to the diet. Many foods rich in polyunsaturated fats also provide other key nutrients. For example, vegetable oils are good sources of vitamin E, and fish and shellfish are rich in high-quality protein and the following vitamins and minerals:

- ▶ Vitamin D—Salmon, mackerel, sardines, and tuna (canned)
- ▶ Potassium—Halibut, haddock, salmon (sockeye), and clams
- ▶ Iron—Clams, oysters, and sardines
- ▶ Magnesium—Halibut and Pollock
- ▶ Calcium—Sardines, pink salmon, ocean perch (Atlantic), blue crab, clams, and rainbow trout

◀ *SEE ALSO 3.3, "Animal Sources of Protein"* ▶

◀ *SEE ALSO Chapter 4, "Vitamins"* ▶

◀ *SEE ALSO Chapter 5, "Minerals"* ▶

Several studies show that replacing saturated fats with foods rich in polyunsaturated and monounsaturated fats without increasing total calories can lower bad LDL cholesterol levels and help prevent heart disease and stroke.

◀ *SEE ALSO 2.2, "Monounsaturated Fats"* ▶

◀ *SEE ALSO 8.1, "Cardiovascular Disease"* ▶

Omega-3 fats have been found to confer some important health benefits. EPA and DHA, the omega-3 fats found in fish, support important functions in the brain, blood vessels, and the immune system. Studies suggest that EPA and DHA might reduce the risk of cardiovascular disease, diabetes, and prostate cancer. There's evidence that consuming about 1 gram of EPA or DHA from supplements or fish can decrease the risk of death from cardiac events in people who have heart disease.

◀ *SEE ALSO Chapter 8, "Eat to Beat Disease"* ▶

EPA and DHA can also protect your eyes from **macular degeneration,** support visual and neurological development in infants (the omega-6 fat arachidonic acid is also believed to play a role in this), and protect against preterm birth.

Some countries recommend lowering intakes of linoleic acid (an omega 6 fat) because they believe that high intakes can negate the benefits of EPA and DHA and increase the risk of inflammatory, immune, or other diseases and conditions. Americans currently consume more than 10 times as much omega-6 fats as omega-3 fats. Although no expert recommendation to reduce linoleic acid has been made in the United States, it's prudent to follow the healthy eating guidelines as outlined by MyPyramid, and to increase omega-3 fats by consuming more fish to boost nutrient intake and improve the overall quality of the diet.

◀ SEE ALSO 2.7, *"Daily Fat and Cholesterol Recommendations"* ▶

◀ SEE ALSO 6.2, *"Your Daily Meal Pattern"* ▶

As with all fat (no matter what types of fatty acids they contain), too much can contribute to excess calorie intake and increase the risk for obesity or being overweight and related diseases and conditions.

◀ SEE ALSO Chapter 8, *"Eat to Beat Disease"* ▶

◀ SEE ALSO Chapter 7, *"Weight Management"* ▶

WORDS TO GO . . . WORDS TO GO . . . WORDS TO GO

Macular degeneration is the progressive deterioration of the macula (the back part of the retina) that can cause blindness.

2.4 | SATURATED FATS

Definition and Dietary Sources

Health Implications

In this subchapter, you learn what saturated fats are and where they're found in the diet. You also learn why consuming too much saturated fat can be harmful.

Definition and Dietary Sources

Saturated fats are usually solid or waxy at room temperature. Foods contain a mix of various types of the following saturated fats: lauric acid, myristic acid, palmitic acid, and stearic acid.

Animal-derived foods and some plant foods are rich sources of saturated fats. Here are some examples of foods high in saturated fat from each category:

▶ Animal foods—Fatty beef, lamb, pork, poultry with skin, beef fat (tallow), lard, cream, butter, cheese, ice cream, and foods made with animal fats (including many baked foods and fried foods)

▶ Plant foods—Coconut, coconut oil, palm oil, palm kernel oil, cocoa butter, palm, and foods made with these

Although saturated fats are found in various combinations in foods, here are some specific saturated fats and their main food sources:

▶ Lauric acid—Coconut oil

▶ Myristic acid—Palm kernel and coconut oils

▶ Palmitic acid—Most fats and oils

▶ Stearic acid—Most fats and oils, cocoa butter, chocolate, and **fully hydrogenated** vegetable **oils**

The following foods represent the top sources of saturated fat in the American diet; the percentage of total saturated fat intake each food represents is also included.

TOP SOURCES OF SATURATED FAT IN THE U.S. DIET

Food Group	Percent of Total Sat. Fat Intake
Cheese	13.1
Beef	11.7
Milk	7.8
Oils	4.9
Ice cream/sherbet/frozen yogurt	4.7
Cakes/cookies/quick breads/ doughnuts	4.7
Butter	4.6
Other fats (shortening and animal fats)	4.4
Salad dressings/mayonnaise	3.7
Poultry	3.6
Margarine	3.2
Sausage	3.1
Potato chips/corn chips/popcorn	2.9
Yeast bread	2.3
Eggs	2.3
Candy	2.0
Hot dogs	<2.0
Cold cuts (excluding ham)	>1.0
Pork (fresh, unprocessed)	>1.0
Cream	>1.0
Bacon	>1.0
Nuts/seeds	>1.0
Pies/crisps/cobblers	>1.0
Cream substitute	>1.0
Ham	>1.0

Source: Cotton et al., Journal of the American Dietetic Association, *2004.*

Health Implications

Too much saturated fat in the diet can raise total cholesterol and bad low-density lipoprotein (LDL) cholesterol levels. Too much cholesterol in the blood can lead to deposits in artery walls that make it tough for blood to flow through to the heart and brain. This can increase risk of heart attack or stroke.

◄ *SEE ALSO 8.1, "Cardiovascular Disease"* ►

Not all saturated fats are created equal; some are more harmful than others. Consider this:

▶ Lauric acid and myristic acid raise blood cholesterol much more than palmitic acid.

▶ Stearic acid has little effect on total, LDL, and HDL cholesterol levels; when consumed, it's converted to oleic acid, a monounsaturated fat that can have a positive effect on blood cholesterol.

◀ *SEE ALSO 2.2, "Monounsaturated Fats"* ▶

Some studies also show that **interesterified oils** (listed as high-stearate, stearic-rich, or interesterified fats on food labels), which are increasingly being used to replace trans fats in many processed and packaged foods, can raise blood cholesterol levels (though not as much as trans fats do) and blood sugar levels.

◀ *SEE ALSO 2.5, "Trans Fats"* ▶

◀ *SEE ALSO 10.1, "Reading Food Labels"* ▶

Choosing mostly lean cuts of meat and poultry instead of fattier ones, vegetable oils instead of solid fats like butter, and low-fat or nonfat dairy products can help you decrease your saturated fat intake and improve your overall dietary pattern. It can even help you curb your calorie intake and help you manage your weight or lose weight if you need to.

◀ *SEE ALSO Chapter 6, "Creating a Daily Meal Plan"* ▶

◀ *SEE ALSO 6.6, "Meat and Beans"* ▶

◀ *SEE ALSO 6.7, "Milk"* ▶

WORDS TO GO . . . WORDS TO GO . . . WORDS TO GO

Fully hydrogenated oils are saturated fats that are made when liquid vegetable oils rich in unsaturated fat are turned into more solid fats by adding hydrogen molecules. These oils are used to create margarines and baked products and are used in cooking. Unlike partially hydrogenated oils, fully hydrogenated oils do not contain any trans fats.

Interesterified oils are chemically or enzymatically altered to create more solid fats; for example, an oil rich in saturated fats (palm oil or a fully hydrogenated oil) is blended with an edible liquid oil to create margarines or shortening. The resulting oils do not contain trans fats.

2.5 TRANS FATS

Definition and Dietary Sources

Health Implications

In this subchapter, you learn what trans fats are and which foods contain a lot of trans fats. You also learn why it's important to keep your intake of trans fats as low as possible.

Definition and Dietary Sources

Trans fats can be monounsaturated or polyunsaturated fats; however, they are structured differently than the other monounsaturated or polyunsaturated fats, which makes them act more like solid or saturated fats.

◀ *SEE ALSO 2.2, "Monounsaturated Fats"* ▶

The two main types in the diet are artificial or industrial and naturally occurring trans fats.

Artificial or industrial trans fats are found in **partially hydrogenated oils** and foods made with or fried in them; these include margarines, commercially baked goods, snack foods, and french fries. Elaidic acid is the primary trans fat found in partially hydrogenated vegetable oils, as the trans form of oleic acid, mono-unsaturated fat.

Naturally occurring trans fats are found in the stomachs of cows, sheep, and goats. In foods, they're found in small amounts in beef, pork, lamb, and butterfat (used to make butter and milk). Vaccenic acid is the trans fat found in meat and butterfat.

Although trans fats are being phased out in the food supply, they're still found in a variety of foods. An estimated 40 percent of trans fat intake in the United States comes from baked goods such as cakes, cookies, crackers, pies, and breads. The following foods are other top contributors to our daily trans fat intake, listed in descending contributing order:

▶ Animal products

▶ Margarine

▶ Fried potatoes

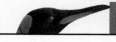

▶ Potato chips, corn chips, popcorn

▶ Household shortening

▶ Breakfast cereal

▶ Candy

Health Implications

Studies have shown that trans fats not only raise total cholesterol and bad LDL cholesterol levels the way saturated fats do, but there is evidence they have further harmful effects by lowering good HDL cholesterol levels. High intakes of trans fats are associated with an increased risk of coronary artery disease, death from coronary heart disease, risk of heart attack, sudden death, and other risk factors for coronary heart disease.

◀ *SEE ALSO 2.4, "Saturated Fats"* ▶

◀ *SEE ALSO 8.1, "Cardiovascular Disease"* ▶

Although the data is limited, recent studies suggest that naturally occurring trans fats don't adversely affect blood cholesterol levels the way man-made trans fats do and therefore might not have the same negative heart-health effects.

Consuming too much trans fat can also mean you're taking in more calories than you need, which can contribute to weight gain and other negative health effects. Too much trans fat can also leave fewer calories available for healthful foods such as fruits, vegetables, and whole grains.

The MyPyramid food guidance system, based on the Dietary Guidelines for Americans, recommends that when we make food and beverage choices, we should opt for those that are lowest in added fats or sugar. Choosing foods with less added fats (for example, having air-popped popcorn with a little canola oil instead of crackers made with added fats) can help us boost our nutritional intake and save on calories and all types of fats including trans fats.

◀ *SEE ALSO 6.2, "Your Daily Meal Pattern"* ▶

WORDS TO GO . . . WORDS TO GO . . . WORDS TO GO

Partially hydrogenated oils turn a liquid vegetable oil into a more solid, stable fat, creating trans fats in the process; the more hydrogens added during hydration, the more saturated (or solid) the fat becomes. But only partially (not fully) hydrogenated oils contain trans fats.

2.6 DIETARY CHOLESTEROL

Definition and Sources

Health Implications

In this subchapter, you learn about dietary cholesterol and its main sources. You also learn why it's important to limit your intake of dietary cholesterol.

Definition and Sources

Dietary cholesterol is a fatlike substance found only in animal foods such as organ meats, egg yolks, fish and shellfish, beef and poultry, and dairy products. Plant foods do not naturally contain cholesterol.

Here's a list of foods and beverages that contribute the most dietary cholesterol to the American diet:

TOP SOURCES OF DIETARY CHOLESTEROL AMONG U.S. ADULTS

Food Group	% Total Cholesterol Intake
Eggs	29.3
Beef	16.1
Poultry	12.2
Cheese	5.8
Milk	5.0
Fish/shellfish (excluding canned tuna)	3.7
Cakes/cookies/quickbreads/doughnuts	3.3
Pork (fresh, unprocessed)	2.8
Ice cream/sherbet/frozen yogurt	2.5
Sausage	2.0
Ham	<2.0
Butter	>1.0
Ham	>1.0
Cold cuts (excluding ham)	>1.0
Organ meats	>1.0
Hot dogs	>1.0
Salad dressings/mayonnaise	>1.0

Source: Cotton et al., Journal of the American Dietetic Association, *2004.*

You might be surprised to learn that although most foods that are high in cholesterol are also high in total fat and saturated fat, some low-fat foods such as shrimp and squid are also high in cholesterol; other shellfish contain lower amounts of cholesterol. Organ meats contain extremely high levels of cholesterol—3 ounces of beef brain, for example, contains a whopping 1,696 mg cholesterol! Here's an estimate of the cholesterol content of some foods:

2.6

DIETARY CHOLESTEROL AMOUNTS IN FOODS AND BEVERAGES

Food	Cholesterol (in mg)
3 oz. beef kidney	609
3 oz. beef liver	337
1 large egg	212
3 oz. shrimp	129
3 oz. ground beef	76
3 oz. lean beef	73
3 oz. lean pork	73
3 oz. chicken breast	71
3 oz. crabmeat	65
3 oz. lobster meat	61
3 oz. salmon	60
3 oz. hotdog	44
2 oz. halibut	35
1 cup whole milk	34
1 cup cottage cheese (4 percent fat)	32
1 tbsp. butter	31
1 oz. cheddar cheese	30

Source: www.nal.usda.gov/fnic/foodcomp/search/.

Health Implications

Although it might have less of an impact than high intakes of saturated and trans fats, too much dietary cholesterol can increase **serum** or **blood cholesterol** levels. When too much cholesterol builds up in blood vessel walls, it's hard for blood to travel through the body and can cause a **heart attack** or **stroke.** When blood vessels that lead to the heart or brain become blocked, a heart attack or stroke can occur.

◄ *SEE ALSO 8.1, "Cardiovascular Disease"* ►

Some people in particular experience wide swings in their blood cholesterol levels in response to consuming varying amounts of dietary cholesterol. Although there's no test to identify who is sensitive to dietary cholesterol, it's prudent for all of us to limit or reduce our intake of dietary cholesterol.

◀ *SEE ALSO 2.7, Daily Fat and Cholesterol Recommendations* ▶

WORDS TO GO . . .WORDS TO GO . . .WORDS TO GO

Serum or **blood cholesterol** is cholesterol that circulates in the bloodstream. Although most is made by the liver, some is obtained from the diet. Two main types of serum cholesterol include LDL (low-density lipoprotein cholesterol, also known as "bad" cholesterol) and HDL (high-density lipoprotein cholesterol, also known as "good" cholesterol).

Heart attack, also known as myocardial infarction (MI), occurs when blood flow to the heart is blocked.

Stroke, also known as a cerebrovascular accident (CVA), occurs when blood flow to the brain is blocked; this causes brain cells to die because they don't get enough oxygen.

2.7 DAILY FAT AND CHOLESTEROL RECOMMENDATIONS

Total Fat

Monounsaturated Fat

Polyunsaturated Fat

Saturated Fat

Trans Fat

Dietary Cholesterol

In this subchapter, you learn how to figure out how much total fat to aim for each day. You also learn recommended limits for the various fats (including saturated and trans fats) and dietary cholesterol.

Total Fat

The Institute of Medicine's dietary reference intakes (DRIs) recommend acceptable macronutrient distribution ranges (AMDRs) for fat for children and adults. These ranges of daily fat intake (expressed as a percentage of total calorie intake) that provide enough fat to meet individual needs while reducing the risk of chronic disease:

▶ Children from 1 to 3 years old—30–40 percent of total calorie intake from fat

▶ Children from 4 to 18 years old—25–35 percent of total calorie intake from fat

▶ Adults from 19 to 70 years and above—20–35 percent of total calorie intake from fat

◀ SEE ALSO 6.1, *"Estimating Your Daily Calorie Needs"* ▶

The DRIs also recommend specific amounts of total fat (in grams) infants should consume each day; these estimated needs are based on adequate intakes (AIs), average intakes of dietary fat by most healthy infants:

▶ Infants 0 to 6 months—31 grams of fat

▶ Infants 7 to 12 months—30 grams of fat

Monounsaturated Fat

Although there are no specific DRIs for monounsaturated fats, the National Cholesterol Education Program Expert Panel on the Detection, Evaluation, and Treatment of High Blood Cholesterol in Adults (Adult Treatment Panel III) recommend up to 20 percent of total daily calorie intake to come from mono-unsaturated fats.

◀ SEE ALSO 2.2, *"Monounsaturated Fats"* ▶

Polyunsaturated Fat

The Institute of Medicine's DRI recommends a range of intake (expressed as a percentage of total calorie intake) for linoleic acid (an omega-6 PUFA) and alpha linolenic acid (an omega-3 PUFA) for children and adults as follows:

▶ Linoleic acid (LA)—5–10 percent of total calories

▶ Alpha-linolenic acid (ALA)—0.6–1.2 percent of total calories

Here are more specific recommendations, based on AIs, for daily intakes of LA and ALA:

DIETARY REFERENCE INTAKES (DRIs) FOR DAILY INTAKE OF LA AND ALA

Age and Stage	Linoleic Acid (g/day)	Alpha-Linolenic Acid (g/day)
Infants		
0–6 months	4.4	0.5
7–12 months	4.6	0.5
Children		
1–3 years	7	0.7
4–8 years	10	0.9
Males		
9–13 years	12	1.2
14–18 years	16	1.6
19–30 years	17	1.6
31–50 years	17	1.6
51–70 years	14	1.6
> 70 years	14	1.6

Age and Stage	Linoleic Acid (g/day)	Alpha-Linolenic Acid (g/day)
Females		
9–13 years	10	1.0
14–18 years	11	1.1
19–30 years	12	1.1
31–50 years	12	1.1
51–70 years	11	1.1
> 70 years	11	1.1
Pregnancy		
14–18 years	13	1.4
19–30 years	13	1.4
31–50 years	13	1.4
Lactation		
14–18 years	13	1.3
19–30 years	13	1.3
31–50 years	13	1.3

Source: Dietary Reference Intakes from Energy, Carbohydrates, Fiber, Fat, Fatty Acids, Cholesterol, Protein, and Amino Acids (2002/2005); www.nap.edu.

Although there are no specific recommendations for EPA and DHA (the omega-3 fats found in fish), the American Heart Association (AHA) recommends everyone eat at least two fish meals (about 8 ounces cooked) each week, which provides about 500 mg/day EPA and DHA.

Saturated Fat

Dietary Guidelines for Americans and the AHA recommends that Americans should consume less than 10 percent of total calories from saturated fat. The AHA also recommends those with elevated bad LDL cholesterol (> 130 mg/dL) to aim for less than 7 percent of total calories from saturated fat.

◄ *SEE ALSO 8.1, "Cardiovascular Disease"* ►

The following table shows how many grams of saturated fat to aim for each day based on your individual daily calorie intake.

DAILY GOALS FOR SATURATED FAT INTAKE

Calorie Level	Less Than 10 Percent of Total Calories	Less Than 7 Percent of Total Calories
1,000	11 grams	8 grams
1,200	13 grams	9 grams
1,400	16 grams	11 grams
1,600	18 grams	12 grams
1,800	20 grams	14 grams
2,000	22 grams	16 grams
2,200	24 grams	17 grams
2,400	27 grams	19 grams
2,600	29 grams	20 grams

Trans Fat

Although the current Dietary Guidelines for Americans recommend that people limit their intake of trans fats, and the Institute of Medicine's DRIs recommend that trans fat intake should be as low as possible, the AHA has set a firm guideline for daily intake of trans fats. Based on their recent 2006 Dietary Guidelines, the AHA recommends that less than 1 percent of total calories should come from trans fats. That equals 1–3 grams of trans fat a day. Here are individual recommendations based on your daily calorie intake:

▶ If you consume 1,000–1,200 calories a day, consume no more than 1 gram per day.

▶ If you consume 1,400 calories a day, consume no more than 1.5 grams per day.

▶ If you consume 1,600–2,000 calories a day, consume no more than 2 grams per day.

▶ If you consume 2,200–2,400 calories a day, consume no more than 2.5 grams per day.

▶ If you consume 2,600 calories per day, consume no more than 3 grams per day.

Dietary Cholesterol

Dietary cholesterol is not something we need to consume; our bodies produce about 1,000 mg each day to meet our daily needs. Despite this, it would be very difficult for all but those who follow a **vegan diet** to eliminate dietary cholesterol from their diets.

◀ *SEE ALSO 2.6, "Dietary Cholesterol"* ▶

The current Dietary Guidelines for Americans recommend a cholesterol intake of less than 300 mg per day. Less than 200 mg (or even less) is recommended for those with elevated LDL cholesterol level (>130 mg/dL) or those diagnosed with heart disease.

WORDS TO GO . . .WORDS TO GO . . .WORDS TO GO

A **vegan diet** is one that excludes all animal-derived foods (including meats, eggs, dairy products, and foods made with animal fats).

3

PROTEINS

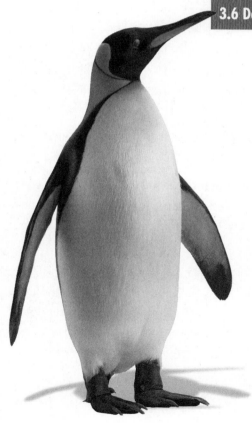

3.1 FUNCTIONS OF PROTEINS

In the Body

In the Diet

Thousands of proteins are found throughout the body. This subchapter covers the many vital roles of proteins both in the body and in the diet.

In the Body

Proteins are found in nearly every body part including muscles, organs, bones, skin, hair, and nails. They provide structural support to the body. For example, collagen is a protein that forms the foundation for bones and teeth, and keratin is a protein found abundantly in hair, nails, and the outer layer of skin. Proteins also help preserve lean muscle tissue that keeps your metabolism revved up, and they support the many important functions of muscles whether they're being used for strenuous exercise or to pump the heart muscle efficiently.

During periods of growth (such as in infancy, childhood, adolescence, and pregnancy), proteins are used by the body to create new tissues. And when our body cells wear down, proteins help rebuild and repair them to help the body function optimally.

Specific types of proteins also help the body work; here are a few examples:

▶ **Enzymes** speed up chemical reactions.

▶ **Antibodies** protect the body from invaders such as bacteria that can cause infection or illness.

▶ **Hemoglobin** helps transport oxygen around the body.

Many **hormones** are also proteins. Hormones send important messages from one part of the body to another. For example, insulin is a hormone released by the pancreas after it detects high levels of glucose (a simple sugar) in the blood. Secreting insulin allows the pancreas to better control blood sugar levels. In insulin-resistance or type 1 or type 2 diabetes, the body can't make any or enough insulin or cannot properly use the insulin it does make to keep blood sugar levels in a healthy range.

◀ SEE ALSO 1.1, *"Functions of Carbohydrates"* ▶

◀ SEE ALSO 8.3, *"Diabetes"* ▶

Several proteins are also responsible for carrying fats, vitamins, minerals, and other substances through the blood to various parts of the body.

In the Diet

Although it's critical to consume adequate amounts of dietary protein each day, we need fewer total calories from protein than we do from carbohydrates and fats—the two other calorie-containing nutrients.

◄ *SEE ALSO 1.5, "Daily Carbohydrate Recommendations"* ▶

◄ *SEE ALSO 2.7, "Daily Fat and Cholesterol Recommendations"* ▶

Unlike carbohydrates and fats, protein cannot be stored in the body; that's why it's important to include protein-rich foods in your diet each day. It's found in a variety of foods from animal and plant sources, including meats, fish, poultry, eggs, dairy products, legumes (beans and peas), soy foods like tofu, nuts, and seeds.

◄ *SEE ALSO 3.3, "Animal Sources of Protein"* ▶

◄ *SEE ALSO 3.4, "Plant Sources of Protein"* ▶

Dietary protein is relatively low in calories. Each gram contains 4 calories, the same amount in 1 gram of carbohydrate. However, studies suggest that protein-rich foods seem to be more satiating or satisfying than foods high in carbohydrates or fats. Plant sources of protein are especially filling because of their high fiber and water content. Consuming many of these foods over time can lower your overall calorie intake and help you achieve or maintain a healthier body weight.

◄ *SEE ALSO Chapter 7, "Weight Management"* ▶

WORDS TO GO . . .WORDS TO GO . . . WORDS TO GO

Enzymes are proteins that speed up chemical reactions.

Antibodies are proteins found in the blood that protect the body from being invaded by bacteria or viruses that can cause illness or infection.

Hemoglobin is the protein in red blood cells; it carries oxygen around the body and brings carbon dioxide to the lungs.

Hormones are proteins that send important messages from one part of the body to another.

3.2 AMINO ACIDS

Definition

Essential vs. Nonessential Amino Acids

In this subchapter, you learn what amino acids are. You also learn about the two types of amino acids and why they're important in the diet and in the body.

Definition

Amino acids are often referred to as the building blocks of proteins. There are 20 amino acids that link together in thousands of ways to form thousands of unique proteins, each with specific functions and roles in the body. When you consume protein-rich foods, the digestive juices in your stomach and intestine break down the protein into amino acids, which are then used to preserve muscles, bones, and organs, and perform other vital functions.

◄ SEE ALSO 3.1, *"Functions of Proteins"* ►

Nonessential vs. Essential Amino Acids

Eleven amino acids are *nonessential*; they're made inside the body in a large enough quantity to meet the body's needs. Nine amino acids are *essential* because the body can't make enough to meet its needs. Here's a list of essential and nonessential amino acids:

AMINO ACIDS

Essential	Nonessential
Histamine	Alanine
Isoleucine	Arginine
Leucine	Asparagine
Lysine	Aspartic acid
Methionine	Cysteine
Phenylalanine	Glutamic acid
Threonine	Glutamine
Tryptophan	Glycine
Valine	Proline
	Serine
	Tyrosine

If you have a rare genetic disorder such as **Phenylketonuria (PKU),** certain metabolic problems, or experience a trauma or critical illness, your body might not be able to make any or enough of the nonessential amino acids it can normally create.

Animal and plant sources of protein vary in their amino acid content. Animal sources of protein are considered complete proteins because they contain all the essential amino acids. On the other hand, most plant sources of protein are considered incomplete proteins because they lack one or more essential amino acids; soybeans are the exception and contain all the essential amino acids. Different plant proteins with different amino acid profiles can be consumed over the course of the day (and not necessarily at each meal as was once believed) to provide the body with more complete, high-quality proteins that can then perform their many vital functions.

◄ *SEE ALSO 3.3, "Animal Sources of Protein"* ►

◄ *SEE ALSO 3.4, "Plant Sources of Protein"* ►

People who are vegans rely on plant foods and consume no animal foods, so they need to consume a variety of plant foods such as soybean products (such as tofu or soy milk), often each day, to get enough essential amino acids.

WORDS TO GO . . .WORDS TO GO . . .WORDS TO GO

Phenylketonuria (PKU) is an inherited disorder caused by a lack or deficiency of the enzyme that converts phenylalanine (an essential amino acid) to tyrosine (a nonessential amino acid).

3.3 ANIMAL SOURCES OF PROTEIN

Overview
Protein Content in Animal Foods

In this subchapter, you learn why foods and beverages derived from animals are important sources of protein for both the diet and the body. You also learn how much protein various animal foods contain.

Overview

Animal foods such as meats, poultry, fish, eggs, and dairy foods supply the body with its best sources of high-quality or **complete proteins.** They contain all the essential amino acids needed by the body to create proteins that perform vital functions.

◀ *SEE ALSO 3.1, "Functions of Proteins"* ▶

Dietary animal protein also provides the body with several vital nutrients, including vitamin B12, folate, biotin, and iron.

◀ *SEE ALSO 4.7, "B Vitamins"* ▶

◀ *SEE ALSO 5.8, "Trace Minerals"* ▶

Some types of fish are excellent sources of eicosapentaenoic acid (EPA) and docosahexaenoic acid (DHA), two essential fats that support brain function and normal growth and development.

◀ *SEE ALSO 2.3, "Polyunsaturated Fats"* ▶

Dairy foods including milk, yogurt, and cheese provide the body with key nutrients such as calcium, phosphorus, and vitamin D.

◀ *SEE ALSO 4.3, "Vitamin D"* ▶

◀ *SEE ALSO 5.5, "Calcium"* ▶

◀ *SEE ALSO 5.6, "Phosphorus"* ▶

Animal sources of protein, including fatty meats, whole-milk dairy products, and eggs, are energy-dense and provide a lot of calories in relatively small portions. They're also high in fat—especially saturated fat—and cholesterol. Too much saturated fat and cholesterol in the diet promotes heart disease. Too many calories from any source can promote weight gain, which also contributes to increased disease risk.

◀ *SEE ALSO 2.4, "Saturated Fats"* ▶

◀ *SEE ALSO 2.6, "Dietary Cholesterol"* ▶

◀ *SEE ALSO 8.1, "Cardiovascular Disease"* ▶

3.3

Choosing appropriate amounts of meat, poultry, fish, milk, and other dairy foods in lean or low-fat forms as recommended by the USDA's MyPyramid can help you reap the full nutritional benefits these foods provide and at the same time minimize harmful saturated fat and dietary cholesterol.

◀ *SEE ALSO 6.6, "Meat and Beans"* ▶

◀ *SEE ALSO 6.7, "Milk"* ▶

Protein Content in Animal Foods

Here's how much dietary protein you'll find in some commonly consumed animal-derived foods and beverages:

AMOUNT OF PROTEIN IN FOODS AND BEVERAGES FROM ANIMAL SOURCES

Food or Beverage	Amount	Protein (g)
Fish, halibut, Atlantic or Pacific, cooked	5½ oz.	43
Fish, salmon, sockeye, cooked	5½ oz.	42
Turkey, meat only, roasted	5	41
Fish, haddock, cooked	5	36
Beef, bottom round, lean	3	29
Cheese, ricotta, part skim	1 cup	28
Cheese, cottage, low-fat, 1% milkfat	1 cup	28
Crustaceans, crab, blue, canned	5 oz.	28
Chicken, broilers or fryers, light meat, cooked	3 oz.	27
Lamb, loin, lean	3 oz.	25
Fish, tuna, yellowfin, fresh, cooked	3 oz.	25
Beef, eye of round, lean	3 oz.	25
Turkey, light meat, roasted	3 oz.	25
Beef, top sirloin, lean, broiled	3 oz.	25

continues

AMOUNT OF PROTEIN IN FOODS AND BEVERAGES
FROM ANIMAL SOURCES (CONTINUED)

Food or Beverage	Amount	Protein (g)
Fish, salmon, sockeye, cooked	3 oz.	23
Pork, fresh, loin, chops, bone in, lean, cooked	3 oz.	23
Fish, halibut, Atlantic and Pacific, cooked	3 oz.	23
Beef, ground, 75% lean/25% fat, patty, cooked	3 oz.	22
Mollusks, clams, canned	3 oz.	22
Fish, tuna, light, canned in water	3 oz.	22
Fish, sardines, Atlantic, canned in oil	3 oz.	21
Fish, tuna, white, canned in water	3 oz.	20
Fish, salmon, pink, canned	3 oz.	17
Cheese, cottage, nonfat	1 cup	15
Yogurt, plain, skim milk	8 fl oz.	13
Yogurt, plain, low-fat	8 fl oz.	12
Ham, sliced, extra lean	2 slices (2 oz.)	11
Milk, fat-free/skim	8 fl oz.	8
Milk, low-fat, 1% milkfat	8 fl oz.	8
Cheese, Swiss	1 oz.	8
Cheese, mozzarella, part skim	1 oz.	7
Egg, whole, hard-boiled	1 large	6
Cheese, processed, American	1 oz.	6

Source: U.S. Department of Agriculture, Agricultural Research Service. 2008. USDA National Nutrient Database for Standard Reference, Release 21. Nutrient Data Laboratory Home Page: www.ars.usda.gov/ba/bhnrc/ndl.

WORDS TO GO . . .WORDS TO GO . . .WORDS TO GO

Complete proteins, also known as high-quality proteins, provide the body with enough of all the essential amino acids (amino acids that need to be provided by dietary sources) to meet the body's needs; these amino acids are then used to make proteins that perform vital functions in the body.

3.4 PLANT SOURCES OF PROTEIN

Overview

Protein Content in Plant Foods

This subchapter covers the various plant sources of protein, including legumes, nuts, and seeds, found in the diet. You learn how the protein in these foods differs from that found in animal sources. You also learn which plant foods are the best sources of dietary protein.

Overview

Protein is found in plant foods including legumes (beans and peas), nuts (and nut butters), and seeds. It's also found to a lesser extent in grains, grain products, and vegetables (both starchy and non-starchy) and in low amounts in fruits. Although soybeans and other soy foods, like all animal sources of protein, contain complete protein, all other plant sources are **incomplete proteins** because they don't contain all the essential amino acids the body needs from dietary sources. Consuming animal sources of protein each day can help you meet your protein needs. If you don't consume these sources, you need to have soy foods and mix up your intake of legumes, nuts, and seeds to help your body get the full array of amino acids it needs.

◀ SEE ALSO 3.2, *"Amino Acids"* ▶

◀ SEE ALSO 3.3, *"Animal Sources of Protein"* ▶

Plant sources of protein also contain a wide array of nutrients such as fiber, vitamins, and minerals. Many are also high in water content and can fill you up, help you lower your overall calorie intake, and manage your weight.

◀ SEE ALSO Chapter 7, *"Weight Management"* ▶

Because some plant foods such as beans, nuts, and nut butters are **energy-dense,** it's wise to have small servings of these foods to maximize nutrients and minimize calorie intake.

◀ SEE ALSO Chapter 6, *"Creating a Daily Meal Plan"* ▶

Legumes

Legumes, including dry beans, peas, lentils, and soybeans, are unique because they're not only rich in protein, but are also a great source of **complex carbohydrates.**

Although most legumes—like most plant foods—are incomplete proteins because they lack one or more amino acids needed by the body, soybeans and soy foods such as tofu, tempeh, and soy milk contain all the **essential amino acids** and are excellent sources of complete or high-quality proteins.

◄ SEE ALSO 3.2, *"Amino Acids"* ▶

Legumes, like all other plant foods, are cholesterol-free and although they do contain some dietary fat, most of it is unsaturated. And some plant foods, including soybeans and soy foods, contain alpha-linolenic acid (ALA), an omega-3 polyunsaturated fatty acid that might lower the risk of heart disease.

Legumes are also a great source of dietary fiber and contain vitamins such as the B vitamin folate and minerals such as potassium, calcium, and magnesium.

◄ SEE ALSO 5.3, *"Potassium"* ▶

◄ SEE ALSO 5.5, *"Calcium"* ▶

MyPyramid recommends ½–3½ cups of legumes each week depending on your individual calorie intake as part of a healthful eating plan to get the many key nutrients and potential health benefits they provide.

◄ SEE ALSO 6.2, *"Your Daily Meal Plan"* ▶

◄ SEE ALSO 6.6, *"Meat and Beans"* ▶

Nuts and Seeds

Nuts, nut butters, and seeds are also good sources of protein, although the protein they contain is incomplete. They also contain high amounts of healthful monounsaturated and polyunsaturated fats. Like soybeans and soy foods, some nuts such as walnuts, flaxseeds, Brazil nuts, hazelnuts, and pecans contain ALA, omega-3 fats that are essential (and must be obtained in the diet).

◄ SEE ALSO 2.2, *"Monounsaturated Fats"* ▶

◄ SEE ALSO 2.3, *"Polyunsaturated Fats"* ▶

Some nuts and seeds are good sources of fiber, vitamins, and minerals. Almonds are high in fiber, while peanuts, which are technically legumes but more similar in nutrients to nuts, are rich in the B vitamin folate. Here are some nuts and seeds that are rich in the following key nutrients:

▶ Vitamin E—Sunflower seed kernals (kernels), almonds, hazelnuts, pine nuts, peanut butter, peanuts, and Brazil nuts

▶ Magnesium—Brazil nuts, almonds, cashews, pine nuts, peanuts, chestnuts, and hazelnuts

◀ SEE ALSO 1.4, *"Dietary Fiber"* ▶

◀ SEE ALSO 4.4, *"Vitamin E"* ▶

◀ SEE ALSO 4.7, *"B Vitamins"* ▶

◀ SEE ALSO 5.7, *"Magnesium"* ▶

Many nuts and seeds—especially walnuts, pecans, and chestnuts—are rich in phytochemicals (many that act as **antioxidants**) such as flavonoids, resveratrol, polyphenols, and tocopherols.

Studies show nuts and seeds might benefit health by:

▶ Reducing the risk of and death from cardiovascular disease

▶ Reducing inflammation that can contribute to many diseases

▶ Reducing the risk of type 2 diabetes

▶ Reducing total cholesterol and bad LDL cholesterol

▶ Regulating body weight (by suppressing appetite and fat absorption)

▶ Reducing the risk of some cancers

◀ SEE ALSO Chapter 7, *"Weight Management"* ▶

◀ SEE ALSO Chapter 8, *"Eat to Beat Disease"* ▶

Protein Content in Plant Foods

The following table shows how much dietary protein you'll find in some commonly consumed plant foods.

AMOUNT OF PROTEIN IN FOODS AND BEVERAGES
FROM PLANT SOURCES

Food or Beverage	Amount	Protein (g)
Soybeans, mature, boiled	1 cup	29
Soybeans, green, boiled	1 cup	22
Beans, white, mature seeds, canned	1 cup	19
Lentils, mature seeds, boiled	1 cup	18
Peas, split, mature seeds, boiled	1 cup	16
Beans, pinto, mature seeds, boiled	1 cup	15
Beans, kidney, red, mature seeds, boiled	1 cup	15
Beans, black, mature seeds, boiled	1 cup	15
Beans, navy, mature seeds, cooked	1 cup	15
Lima beans, large, mature seeds, boiled	1 cup	15
Chickpeas (garbanzo beans, bengal gram), mature seeds, cooked	1 cup	15
Refried beans, canned	1 cup	14
Baked beans, plain or vegetarian, canned	1 cup	12
Tofu, soft, prepared with calcium sulfate and magnesium chloride (nigari)	1 piece (4 oz.)	8
Peanuts, dry roasted	28	7
Tofu, firm, prepared with calcium sulfate and magnesium chloride (nigari)	¼ block (3 oz.)	7
Wild rice, cooked	1 cup	7
Sunflower seeds, dry roasted	¼ cup	6
Nuts, pistachio, dry roasted	47 (1 oz.)	6
Nuts, almonds	24 (1 oz.)	6
Couscous, cooked	1 cup	6
Cereals, oats, cooked	1 cup	6
Bulgur, cooked	1 cup	6
Peas, edible-podded, boiled	1 cup	5
Potato, baked	1 (7 oz.)	5
Rice, brown, cooked	1 cup	5

Source: U.S. Department of Agriculture, Agricultural Research Service. 2008. USDA National Nutrient Database for Standard Reference, Release 21. Nutrient Data Laboratory Home Page: www.ars.usda.gov/ba/bhnrc/ndl.

Incomplete proteins are proteins that lack one or more **essential amino acids** (amino acids that are needed from dietary sources); without all these essential amino acids, the body is unable to create all the proteins it needs to perform vital functions.

An **energy-dense** food or beverage has a high level of calories per volume.

Complex carbohydrates are carbohydrates made of more than two monosaccharides (single sugar units); starches and fibers are complex carbohydrates.

Antioxidants are substances that protect the body against free radicals, unstable molecules that attack body cells.

3.4

3.5 DEFICIENCIES AND EXCESSES OF PROTEIN

Deficiencies
Excesses

In this subchapter, you learn the potential consequences of consuming too little or too much dietary protein.

Deficiencies

Although protein deficiencies are prevalent in certain populations around the world, they're not very common in the United States where many of us consume a lot more protein than typically recommended. However, some of the following people might be at risk for not getting enough protein to meet their needs:

▶ Those who don't consume enough total calories, either because of poverty or an eating disorder such as anorexia

▶ Older Americans who might consume fewer total calories and/or have trouble chewing meats and other tough protein-rich foods

▶ Those who follow vegetarian or vegan diets and don't get enough high-quality protein

▶ Those who have a disease or chronic illness that makes it difficult for them to consume adequate amounts of nutrient-rich foods

If you don't consume enough protein-rich foods each day, you won't get enough of the essential amino acids you need to make body proteins that support the growth and maintenance of body tissues among other functions. Even if you do consume enough total protein, unless you're consuming adequate amounts of foods that are rich in high-quality protein (including animal-derived foods and soy foods), your diet might fall short on essential amino acids.

◀ SEE ALSO 3.1, *"Functions of Proteins"* ▶

◀ SEE ALSO 3.2, *"Amino Acids"* ▶

Getting inadequate amounts of protein can be especially damaging to older people. As we age, our body composition shifts; we lose muscle mass and accumulate more body fat. Too little dietary protein can degrade body proteins even more, which means the body is less able to heal wounds and fractures and

fight infections. Muscles might also feel weaker, which can make it more difficult to move and increase the risk of falling. Some experts believe the recommended dietary allowance (RDA) for protein for older people should be raised by 25 percent to 1.0 gram per kilogram of body weight.

◀ *SEE ALSO 3.6, "Daily Protein Recommendations"* ▶

Another consequence of inadequate protein intake (when overall calorie intake is also insufficient to meet daily needs) is that the body compensates by breaking down its own body proteins to create energy in the form of glucose—the main fuel source for the brain, lungs, and entire nervous system. This prevents body proteins from doing the important jobs they're meant to do.

◀ *SEE ALSO 1.1, "Functions of Carbohydrates"* ▶

◀ *SEE ALSO 8.1, "Cardiovascular Disease"* ▶

Over time, too little protein and/or too few calories can cause **protein-energy malnutrition (PEM)**. Two severe types of PEM include

▶ Kwashiorkor—Kwashiorkor is malnutrition caused by inadequate consumption of dietary protein, often in impoverished countries. Symptoms include poor growth, weakness, apathy, edema, and increased risk for infection.

▶ Marasmus—Marasmus is malnutrition caused by consuming too little protein and too few calories. Muscle, fat, and other body tissues break down to create energy for the body. Other symptoms include weight loss and impaired immune function. Marasmus can occur in people who have malabsorption or kidney problems.

Excesses

Too much dietary protein can strain the kidneys, whose job is to remove wastes from the blood, among other important functions. Excess protein can also cause bones to excrete calcium, which can increase the risk of bone loss and osteoporosis.

◀ *SEE ALSO 8.6, "Osteoporosis"* ▶

Consuming more dietary protein than you need—especially from high-calorie sources—can lead to excess total calorie intake. The body will take that extra protein, break it down, and store it as body fat.

Too many protein-rich animal foods, including fatty meats and whole milk dairy products, can contribute too much total fat, saturated fat, and cholesterol to the diet. This can increase the risk for developing cardiovascular disease, high blood cholesterol, hypertension, and other conditions.

◀ *SEE ALSO 3.3, "Animal Sources of Protein"* ▶

◀ *SEE ALSO 8.1, "Cardiovascular Disease"* ▶

◀ *SEE ALSO 8.2, "Hypertension"* ▶

Too many protein-rich foods might also leave less room in the diet for nutrient-dense food choices such as fruits, vegetables, and whole grains. If you have too many high-protein foods at the expense of these, you might consume less total fiber and lower amounts of the vitamins, minerals, and other beneficial substances these plant foods provide.

◀ *SEE ALSO Chapter 6, "Creating a Daily Meal Plan"* ▶

WORDS TO GO . . . WORDS TO GO . . . WORDS TO GO

Protein-energy malnutrition (PEM) is a condition that results from inadequate intake of dietary protein and energy (measured as calories) over a long period of time. It can lead to the breakdown of body tissues (including muscle tissue) and increase the risk of infection.

3.6   DAILY PROTEIN RECOMMENDATIONS

Acceptable Macronutrient Distribution Range for Protein

Recommended Dietary Allowance for Protein

This subchapter shows you how to determine how much protein to aim for each day based on your individual needs.

Acceptable Macronutrient Distribution Range for Protein

The Food and Nutrition Board of the Institute of Medicine created acceptable macronutrient distribution ranges (AMDRs) for protein as well as the other key nutrients (carbohydrate and fat) that provide the body with energy. It recommends that 10–35 percent of total calories should come from dietary protein.

◀ *SEE ALSO 1.5, "Daily Carbohydrate Recommendations"* ▶

◀ *SEE ALSO 2.7, "Daily Fat and Cholesterol Recommendations"* ▶

Here's how someone can determine his ideal range for protein intake (in calories) each day based on the AMDR:

1. Multiply total daily calories by 0.10 (percent of total calories).

2. Take the answer from #1 and divide by 4 (calories per gram) to get the number of grams.

3. Multiply total daily calories by 0.35 (percent of total calories) to get number of grams.

4. Take the answer from #3 and divide by 4 calories per gram.

5. Your daily range of intake should be between the answer from #2 and the answer from #4.

◀ *SEE ALSO 6.1, "Estimating Your Daily Calorie Needs"* ▶

For example, if you consume 2,000 calories a day, here's how you would figure your range of daily protein intake:

1. 2,000 multiplied by 0.10 equals 200 calories.

2. 200 calories divided by 4 calories per gram equals 50 grams.

3. 2,000 multiplied by 0.35 equals 700 calories.

4. 700 calories divided by 4 calories per gram equals 175 grams.

5. This person should aim for 50–175 grams of protein each day.

◀ *SEE ALSO 3.3, "Animal Sources of Protein"* ▶

◀ *SEE ALSO 3.4, "Plant Sources of Protein"* ▶

Recommended Dietary Allowances for Protein

More specific daily protein recommendations are provided by the RDAs. These were created to help most people meet their individual needs. The RDA for protein assumes that the dietary pattern provides enough calories and key nutrients to prevent proteins from being used to create energy and instead allow them to be used to perform their many functions.

◀ *SEE ALSO 3.1, "Functions of Proteins"* ▶

You can use the following table to determine your individual daily protein needs.

DAILY RECOMMENDATIONS FOR DIETARY PROTEIN INTAKE

Age	RDA (in grams)	Age	RDA (in grams)
Infants		**Males**	
0–6 months	9.1*	14–18 years	52
7–12 months	11	19–70+ years	56
Children		**Females**	
1–3 years	13	14–18 years	46
4–8 years	19	19–70+ years	46
9–13 years	34	Pregnancy	71
14–18 years	46	Lactation	71

This value is not an RDA but an adequate intake (AI) level designed to cover the needs of all individuals in the group (although there's not enough data to say which percentage of that group is covered).

Source: Dietary Reference Intakes for Energy, Carbohydrate, Fiber, Fat, Fatty Acids, Cholesterol, Protein, and Amino Acids (2002/2005).

Here are intake recommendations for protein based on actual body weight and age (in clinical situations, **ideal body weight** might be used to determine daily protein needs):

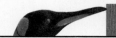

DAILY RECOMMENDATIONS FOR DIETARY PROTEIN INTAKE

Age	RDA (grams/kilogram)	Age	RDA (grams/kilogram)
0–6 months	1.52	9–13 years	0.95
7–12 months	1.2	14–18 years	0.85
1–3 years	1.05	19+ years	0.8
4–8 years	0.95		

Source: Dietary Reference Intakes for Energy, Carbohydrate, Fiber, Fat, Fatty Acids, Cholesterol, Protein, and Amino Acids (2002/2005).

3.6

To determine how this translates into grams of protein, do the following:

1. Take your weight (in pounds) and divide that number by 2.205 kilograms per pound. That's how many kilograms you weigh.

2. Take the answer from number 1 and multiply that by 0.8. That's an estimate for how many grams of protein to aim for each day.

If, for example, you are a 40-year-old adult female (who is not pregnant or lactating) and you weigh about 110 pounds, here's how you'd do the math:

1. 110 pounds divided by 2.205 kilograms per pound equals about 50 kilograms.

2. 50 kilograms multiplied by 0.8 grams per kilogram equals about 40 grams.

WORDS TO GO . . . *WORDS TO GO . . .WORDS TO GO*

Ideal body weight is a desirable and healthful weight range based on height.

4

VITAMINS

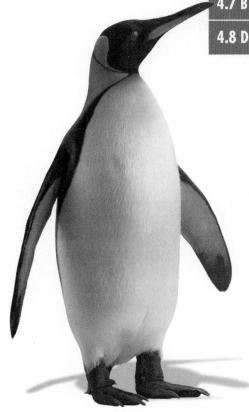

4.1   FUNCTIONS OF VITAMINS

Overview

Classes

In this subchapter, you learn why vitamins are so important in the body. You also learn about the two classes of vitamins found in the diet and in the body.

Overview

Your body needs small amounts of vitamins to help it grow, develop, and function properly. Although vitamins are **micronutrients** and don't provide calories or energy to the body the way the **macronutrients** (carbohydrates, fats, and proteins) do, they perform many vital functions to help the body operate smoothly and efficiently.

◄ SEE ALSO 1.1, *"Functions of Carbohydrates"* ▷

◄ SEE ALSO 2.1, *"Functions of Fats"* ▷

◄ SEE ALSO 3.1, *"Functions of Proteins"* ▷

Most of us can usually get all the vitamins we need by consuming a nutrient-dense, well-balanced diet that incorporates all the key food groups. Our bodies can also make two vitamins—D and K—to help us meet our daily needs. Nevertheless, there are some times in life and some situations during which vitamin supplements might be warranted. Those who might need specific vitamin supplements include the following:

▶ People who follow vegetarian diets might need a vitamin B12 supplement if they don't consume many animal products. Vegans definitely need a B12 supplement, as it is not found in plant foods.

▶ Women who are planning to become pregnant are urged to take a folic acid supplement.

▶ Older people, who have a lower ability to absorb vitamin B12 because of declining stomach acidity with age, could benefit from a multivitamin that includes it.

◄ SEE ALSO 4.7, *"B Vitamins"* ▷

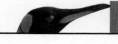

▶ Those who follow limited or special diets because of food allergies, sensitivities, or certain medical conditions might need a multivitamin supplement.

◀ *SEE ALSO Chapter 8, "Eat to Beat Disease"* ▶

◀ *SEE ALSO Chapter 9, "Food Allergies, Intolerances, and Sensitivities"* ▶

Classes

There are 13 vitamins; they are categorized as either fat-soluble or water-soluble.

Fat-Soluble Vitamins

Fat-soluble vitamins dissolve in fat tissue before they're absorbed by the bloodstream and can perform their vital functions. If you consume more of them than is required, the excesses are stored in the liver.

4.1

The fat-soluble vitamins are vitamins A, D, E, and K. Vitamin A helps eyes and skin stay healthy and protects the body against infections. Vitamin D helps the body absorb calcium and can protect against several diseases, including colon cancer. Vitamin E acts as an antioxidant to protect vitamin A and essential fatty acids against harmful substances that can destroy them. Vitamin K helps blood clot, and there is increasing evidence it helps keeps bones strong, may help keep inflammation at bay, and may have a role in controlling blood glucose levels.

Fat-soluble vitamins are not needed by the body every day because they can be stored for long periods of time in the liver and fatty tissues for use when needed.

Water-Soluble Vitamins

Water-soluble vitamins dissolve in water and are eliminated by the body because they cannot be stored. They include eight B vitamins (thiamine, riboflavin, niacin, pantothenic acid, biotin, folate, vitamin B6, and vitamin B12) and vitamin C. B vitamins play a key role in **metabolism** and help the body release energy from carbohydrates, fat, and protein; vitamin C helps heal cuts and wounds, keeps teeth and gums healthy, and oversees the growth and repair of all body tissues.

Micronutrients are essential nutrients such as vitamins and minerals that are required in relatively small amounts by the body to help you grow and stay healthy.

Macronutrients are essential nutrients such as carbohydrates, fats, and proteins that are required in relatively large amounts to help you grow and stay healthy.

Metabolism is a set of chemical reactions that occur in the body to support normal growth and development, assist reproduction, and maintain structures. Metabolism includes anabolism (building up complex substances from simpler molecules) and catabolism (breaking down complex substances into simpler molecules).

4.2 VITAMIN A

Functions

Dietary Sources

Deficiencies and Excesses

This subchapter covers the key functions and top food sources of vitamin A. It also discusses the effects of getting too little or too much vitamin A.

Functions

Vitamin A is a fat-soluble vitamin that performs several key functions in the body:

4.2

- ▶ Helps create and maintain healthy teeth, bones, and soft tissues in the body

- ▶ Preserves your skin and mucous membranes so they can protect your body from being invaded by bacteria or viruses that can cause an illness or infection

- ▶ Helps create pigments found in the retina of the eye and helps you see, especially at night

- ▶ Supports reproduction, the development of an embryo, and breastfeeding

- ▶ Regulates and strengthens the immune system

- ▶ Acts as an antioxidant to protect cells against damage from free radicals that can contribute to some chronic diseases and unhealthy aging

Dietary Sources

The two main dietary sources of vitamin A are retinol (preformed vitamin A) and Provitamin A carotenoids.

Retinol, the active or usable form of vitamin A, is found most abundantly in animal foods such as meats and dairy products. The vitamin A from animal foods, also called *preformed* vitamin A, is better absorbed and used by the body than the vitamin A in plant foods.

Provitamin A carotenoids are orange pigments found in fruits, vegetables, and other plant foods that can be converted in the body (liver) into usable retinol. Beta-carotene, alpha-carotene, and beta-cryptoxanthin are provitamin A carotenoids commonly found in plant foods. Although all these become retinol in the body, beta-carotene is much more efficiently converted than the other carotenoids. Key food sources of beta-carotene include deeply colored fruits and vegetables such as cantaloupe, pink grapefruit, apricots, pumpkin, carrots, sweet potatoes, winter squash, broccoli, spinach, and most dark green leafy vegetables.

Vitamin A recommendations are sometimes expressed as retinol activity equivalents (RAE); this unit of measuring the vitamin A in foods is useful because it reflects the differences in conversion to vitamin A between animal and plant sources of vitamin A. One RAE equals:

▶ 1 microgram (mcg) retinol

▶ 12 micrograms (mcg) beta-carotene

Vitamin A is expressed as international units (IUs) on food labels and on supplement packages. One IU of preformed vitamin A equals 3.33 IU.

The following table shows food sources that are good or excellent sources of vitamin A based on the current **daily value,** expressed in IUs, for vitamin A.

FOOD SOURCES OF VITAMIN A THAT PROVIDE AT LEAST 10 PERCENT OF THE DAILY VALUE (5000 INTERNATIONAL UNITS) OF VITAMIN A (LISTED IN DESCENDING ORDER)

Food	Amount	Vit. A (IU)
Carrot juice, canned	1 cup	45,132.6
Sweet potato, cooked, baked	1 cup	28,058.3
Carrots, cooked, boiled	1 cup	26,571.5
Beef, variety meats and byproducts, liver	3 oz.	22,174.8
Collards, frozen	1 cup	19,538.1
Kale, cooked, boiled	1 cup	17,707.3
Beet greens, boiled	1 cup	11,021.8
Squash, winter, all types, cooked	1 cup	10,707.2
Mustard greens, cooked	1 cup	8,852.2
Cabbage, Chinese (bok choy), cooked	1 cup	7,223.3
Melons, cantaloupe, raw	1 cup	5,411.2
Lettuce, romaine, raw	1 cup	4,877.6
Peppers, sweet, red, raw	1 cup	4,665.2
Apricots, canned, juice packed, with skin	1 cup	4,126.0
Papayas, raw	1	3,325.8
Spinach, raw	1 cup	2,813.1
Malted drink mix, chocolate	3 tsp.	2,750.6

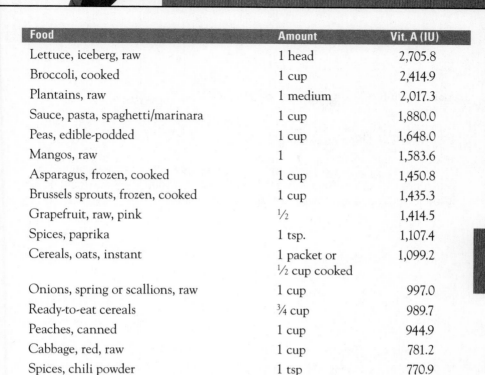

Food	Amount	Vit. A (IU)
Lettuce, iceberg, raw	1 head	2,705.8
Broccoli, cooked	1 cup	2,414.9
Plantains, raw	1 medium	2,017.3
Sauce, pasta, spaghetti/marinara	1 cup	1,880.0
Peas, edible-podded	1 cup	1,648.0
Mangos, raw	1	1,583.6
Asparagus, frozen, cooked	1 cup	1,450.8
Brussels sprouts, frozen, cooked	1 cup	1,435.3
Grapefruit, raw, pink	½	1,414.5
Spices, paprika	1 tsp.	1,107.4
Cereals, oats, instant	1 packet or ½ cup cooked	1,099.2
Onions, spring or scallions, raw	1 cup	997.0
Ready-to-eat cereals	¾ cup	989.7
Peaches, canned	1 cup	944.9
Cabbage, red, raw	1 cup	781.2
Spices, chili powder	1 tsp	770.9

Source: U.S. Department of Agriculture, Agricultural Research Service. 2008. USDA National Nutrient Database for Standard Reference, Release 21. Nutrient Data Laboratory Home Page, www.ars.usda.gov/ba/bhnrc/ndl.

◀ SEE ALSO 4.8, *"Daily Vitamin Recommendations"* ▶

Deficiencies and Excesses

Vitamin A is considered a nutrient of concern for both children and adults according to the 2005 Dietary Guidelines Advisory Committee Report. Although it's rare to be deficient in vitamin A, symptoms can include night blindness or dry, rough skin. Lower resistance to infections, impaired tooth development, and slower bone growth can also occur.

Too much vitamin A from foods and/or supplements can cause nausea, irritability, and blurred vision. Excessive amounts can cause growth retardation, liver problems, hair loss, and bone pain. Large amounts of carotenoids can cause your skin to turn yellow or orange, but this is not harmful and is reversed once you cut back on whatever you are eating that is rich in carotenoids (often, carrots). It can also increase the risk for bone fractures and osteoporosis. Those who consume high amounts of alcohol, have liver disease or high blood cholesterol levels, or consume little dietary protein can be at increased risk for these effects.

◀ *SEE ALSO 10.3 "Functional Foods"* ▶

◀ *SEE ALSO 10.5, "Dietary Supplements"* ▶

◀ *SEE ALSO 8.6, "Osteoporosis"* ▶

WORDS TO GO . . .WORDS TO GO . . .WORDS TO GO

Daily Value (DV) is a dietary reference value for adults of all ages and both sexes that appears on food labels to help Americans compare the amount of nutrients in products in the context of their total diet.

4.3   VITAMIN D

Functions

Sources

Deficiencies and Excesses

This subchapter covers the key functions and top food sources of vitamin D. It also discusses the potential effects of getting too little or too much vitamin D.

Functions

Vitamin D is a fat-soluble vitamin that helps control the level of calcium and phosphorus in the blood to help the body build and maintain strong bones and teeth. It also helps increase the body's absorption of calcium.

◀ *SEE ALSO 5.5, "Calcium"* ▶

◀ *SEE ALSO 5.6, "Phosphorus"* ▶

Recent research suggests that getting adequate amounts of vitamin D (even more than currently recommended) can help protect against osteoporosis, hypertension, cancer, and autoimmune diseases.

Sources

The two main sources of vitamin D include the diet and sunlight.

Dietary

Vitamin D is found naturally in only a few foods, most notably in fish. Most vitamin D we consume, however, comes from fortified foods including milk, margarine, and ready-to-eat cereal. Following is a list of foods that are good or excellent sources of vitamin D.

FOOD SOURCES THAT PROVIDE AT LEAST 10 PERCENT OF THE DAILY VALUE (400 INTERNATIONAL UNITS) OF VITAMIN D (LISTED IN DESCENDING ORDER)

Food	Amount	Vit. D (IU)
Cod liver oil	1 tbsp	1,360
Salmon, cooked	3½ oz.	360
Mackerel, cooked	3½ oz.	345

continues

**FOOD SOURCES THAT PROVIDE AT LEAST 10 PERCENT
OF THE DAILY VALUE (400 INTERNATIONAL UNITS)
OF VITAMIN D (LISTED IN DESCENDING ORDER)** (CONTINUED)

Food	Amount	Vit. D (IU)
Sardines, canned in oil, drained	1¾ oz.	250
Tuna fish, canned in oil	3 oz.	200
Milk, nonfat, reduced fat, and whole, fortified	1 cup	98
Margarine, fortified	1 tbsp.	60
Ready-to-eat cereal, fortified	¾ to 1 cup	40
Egg	1	20
Liver, beef, cooked	1	15
Cheese, Swiss	1 oz.	12

Source: Dietary Supplement Fact Sheet: Vitamin D; ods.od.nih.gov/factsheets/vitamind.asp#h3.

◁ *SEE ALSO 4.8, "Daily Vitamin Recommendations"* ▷

◁ *SEE ALSO 10.3, "Functional Foods"* ▷

Sunlight

Vitamin D (in the form of vitamin D3, the kind found in foods) can be made in the body when the skin is exposed to ultraviolet-B (UVB) rays from sunlight for as little as 10 or 15 minutes.

Deficiencies and Excesses

Some people are at high risk for not getting or making enough vitamin D to meet their daily needs. These include

- ▶ Older people
- ▶ People with dark skin
- ▶ Obese people
- ▶ Infants who are exclusively breastfed
- ▶ People who live in environments or climates in which sunlight is limited
- ▶ People with certain conditions that limit absorption of fat, such as **cystic fibrosis** and **Crohn's disease**
- ▶ People who follow vegetarian or vegan diets and avoid fish, fish oils, and D-fortified dairy and other foods like milk and orange juice

Without enough vitamin D, blood levels of calcium and phosphate can get too low, which can cause the body to produce hormones that release calcium and phosphate from the bones, causing bones to soften and weaken. In children, a vitamin D deficiency causes **rickets.** In adults, it causes **osteomalacia.**

Too much vitamin D from supplements can cause symptoms such as nausea, vomiting, decreased appetite and weight loss, weakness, confusion, altered heart rhythm, and calcium and phosphate deposits in soft tissues. However, D toxicity is now believed to be much less likely than previously believed unless intake routinely exceeds the 1,000 to 2,000 IU a day that experts now recommend.

◁ *SEE ALSO 10.5, "Dietary Supplements"* ▷

WORDS TO GO . . .WORDS TO GO . . .WORDS TO GO

4.3

Cystic fibrosis is an inherited disease that causes endocrine glands (organs that make and secrete hormones into the bloodstream) to malfunction. Mucus becomes thick and sticky and damages other body organs and can lead to serious problems with the lungs, pancreas, and digestive system.

Crohn's disease is a lifelong inflammatory bowel disease that causes swelling and ulcers (deep sores) in the intestinal tract.

Rickets is a bone disease that occurs in infants and children who have a vitamin D deficiency; symptoms include soft, bendable bones.

Osteomalacia is a bone disease caused by a vitamin D deficiency in adulthood; bones soften and cause bowed legs and curvature of the spine.

4.4 VITAMIN E

Functions

Dietary Sources

Deficiencies and Excesses

This subchapter discusses the key functions and top food sources of vitamin E. The health effects associated with too much or too little vitamin E are also described.

Functions

Vitamin E is a fat-soluble vitamin that plays an important role as an antioxidant. It protects vitamins A and C, red blood cells, and **essential fatty acids** from being destroyed by free radicals, which are unstable substances in the environment and in the body. Vitamin E also helps form red blood cells and helps the body use vitamin K.

◄ *SEE ALSO Chapter 2, "Fats"* ▶

◄ *SEE ALSO 4.1, "Vitamin A"* ▶

◄ *SEE ALSO 4.5, "Vitamin K"* ▶

◄ *SEE ALSO 4.6, "Vitamin C"* ▶

Vitamin E has also been shown to play a role in immune function and repair of deoxyribonucleic acid (DNA), a set of instructions for our genes.

Vitamin E might also play a role in heart health by preventing oxidation of bad low-density lipoprotein (LDL) cholesterol and unhealthy plaque buildup in coronary arteries.

◄ *SEE ALSO 8.1, "Cardiovascular Disease"* ▶

Dietary Sources

Vitamin E is not found abundantly in the diet, although some foods, including vegetable oils, green leafy vegetables, and nuts are natural sources. Some foods are also fortified with vitamin E.

Vitamin E is listed as IUs on food labels and dietary supplement packages. One milligram (mg) of alpha-tocopherol, the form of vitamin E found abundantly in the body, equals 1.49 IUs.

Here are some foods that are good or excellent sources of vitamin E (expressed as milligrams of alpha-tocopherol):

**FOOD SOURCES THAT PROVIDE AT LEAST
10 PERCENT OF THE DAILY VALUE (22 MILLIGRAMS)
OF VITAMIN E (LISTED IN DESCENDING ORDER)**

Food	Amount	Vit. E (mg)
Ready-to-eat cereals, fortified	1 cup	13.50
Tomato products, canned, paste	1 cup	11.27
Sunflower seed kernels, dry roasted	¼ cup	8.35
Almonds	24 nuts	7.43
Spinach, frozen, cooked	1 cup	6.73
Sauce, pasta, marinara	1 cup	6.00
Sunflower oil	1 tbsp.	5.59
Hazelnuts	1 oz. (20)	4.26

Source: U.S. Department of Agriculture, Agricultural Research Service. 2008. USDA National Nutrient Database for Standard Reference, Release 21. Nutrient Data Laboratory Home Page, www.ars.usda.gov/ba/bhnrc/ndl.

◁ SEE ALSO 4.8, *"Daily Vitamin Recommendations"* ▷

◁ SEE ALSO 10.3, *"Functional Foods"* ▷

Deficiencies and Excesses

Vitamin E deficiency is rare, mostly only among premature infants and people who cannot absorb dietary fat (such as those with cystic fibrosis). They can experience symptoms such as muscle weakness, balance problems, and impaired vision.

Too much vitamin E can decrease the availability of or interfere with the body's use of other fat-soluble vitamins (A, D, and K). Symptoms can include nausea and problems with the digestive tract.

Although the upper limit for vitamin E is 1,000 IU, in 2004, the American Heart Association warned that consuming more than 400 IU of vitamin E from supplements can cause harm and increase death risk.

Those who take blood-thinning medications or statins such as Coumadin should speak with their physician before taking vitamin E supplements because they can interfere with the effectiveness of their medications or be harmful.

◄ *SEE ALSO 10.5, "Dietary Supplements"* ►

WORDS TO GO . . .WORDS TO GO . . .WORDS TO GO

Essential fatty acids are fatty acids the body needs to obtain from the diet because it cannot make any or enough of them to meet the body's needs.

4.5   VITAMIN K

Functions

Sources

Deficiencies and Excesses

In this subchapter, you learn about the key roles of vitamin K and its sources in the diet and in the body. You also learn about vitamin K deficiencies and excesses.

Functions

Vitamin K is a fat-soluble vitamin needed by the liver to help it create several proteins required to help the blood clot. It also supports proteins involved in bone metabolism and cell growth.

Sources

Several foods are rich in vitamin K.

Dietary

Vitamin K is found as phylloquinone (vitamin K1) mostly in plant foods like leafy greens and other vegetables, soybeans, and cereals.

Here are some foods that are good or excellent sources of vitamin K in the diet:

FOOD SOURCES THAT PROVIDE AT LEAST 10 PERCENT OF THE DAILY VALUE (80 MICROGRAMS) OF VITAMIN K (LISTED IN DESCENDING ORDER)

Food	Amount	Vit. K (mcg)
Kale, frozen, cooked	1 cup	1,146.6
Collards, frozen, cooked	1 cup	1,059.4
Spinach, frozen, cooked	1 cup	1,027.3
Spinach, fresh, cooked	1 cup	987.8
Beet greens, cooked	1 cup	697.0
Mustard greens, cooked	1 cup	419.3
Brussels sprouts, frozen, cooked	1 cup	299.9
Broccoli, cooked,	1 cup	220.1
Onions, spring or scallions, raw	1 cup	207.0
Lettuce, butterhead, raw	1 head	166.7

continues

FOOD SOURCES THAT PROVIDE AT LEAST 10 PERCENT OF THE DAILY VALUE (80 MICROGRAMS) OF VITAMIN K (LISTED IN DESCENDING ORDER) (CONTINUED)

Food	Amount	Vit. K (mcg)
Parsley, raw	10 sprigs	164.0
Cabbage, cooked, boiled	1 cup	163.1
Noodles, egg or spinach, cooked, enriched	1 cup	161.8
Beans, red kidney, cooked	1 cup	14.9
Carrots, raw	1 medium	9.5
Buckwheat flour	1 cup	8.4
Soymilk, unfortified	1 cup	7.4
Muffins, oat bran	1 muffin	7.4
Squash, summer, cooked	1 cup	6.3
Sweet potato, baked in skin	1	3.4
Turkey, all classes, cooked	3 oz.	3.3
Beef, variety meats and byproducts, liver, cooked	3 oz.	3.3

Source: U.S. Department of Agriculture, Agricultural Research Service. 2008. USDA National Nutrient Database for Standard Reference, Release 21. Nutrient Data Laboratory Home Page, www.ars.usda.gov/ba/bhnrc/ndl.

◄ *SEE ALSO 4.8, "Daily Vitamin Recommendations"* ►

In the Body

Some vitamin K can be made by bacteria in the intestines, although the amount created is not enough to meet your daily needs.

Deficiencies and Excesses

Because vitamin K, like other fat-soluble vitamins, is stored in the liver, deficiencies are uncommon. They might occur because of inadequate absorption of vitamin K caused by long-term use of antibiotics; blood thinning medications; or conditions such as celiac disease, **ulcerative colitis,** or cystic fibrosis. Those who have chronic diarrhea or are malnourished because of alcoholism or other causes can also become deficient in vitamin K. Signs of a deficiency include increased bruising and bleeding.

Too much vitamin K, though rare, can cause blood clots and promote the breakdown of red blood cells. It can also lead to jaundice.

It's important for those who take Coumadin or other blood thinners to monitor their intake of vitamin K from foods and supplements. The Food and Nutrition Board of the Institute of Medicine recommends getting vitamin K only from food sources, not from vitamin K supplements, to prevent excessive intake. If you regularly take a daily multivitamin that has K in it, be sure your doctor adjusts your Coumadin dose.

◀ *SEE ALSO 10.5, "Dietary Supplements"* ▶

WORDS TO GO . . .WORDS TO GO . . .WORDS TO GO

Ulcerative colitis is an inflammatory bowel disease that causes inflammation and sores in the lining of the rectum and colon; symptoms often include diarrhea.

4.5

4.6 VITAMIN C

Functions

Dietary Sources

Deficiencies and Excesses

In this subchapter, you learn the many vital roles vitamin C, a water-soluble vitamin, plays in the body. You learn which foods and beverages provide the most vitamin C. You also learn the health risks associated with too much or too little vitamin C.

Functions

Vitamin C, also known as ascorbic acid, is a water-soluble vitamin that has many important functions in the body. Vitamin C:

▶ Helps produce collagen, a protein that holds bones and other tissues together

▶ Heals cuts and wounds

▶ Helps maintain bones, teeth, gums, and blood vessels

▶ Helps form and repair red blood cells, bones, and other tissues

▶ Strengthens the immune system

▶ Helps the body absorb iron from plant foods

Dietary Sources

Because vitamin C is not stored in the body, you need to consume vitamin C-rich foods such as citrus fruits each day. Here are some good or excellent sources of vitamin C in the diet:

FOOD SOURCES THAT PROVIDE AT LEAST 10 PERCENT OF THE DAILY VALUE (60 MILLIGRAMS) OF VITAMIN C (LISTED IN DESCENDING ORDER)

Food	Amount	Vit. C (mg)
Orange juice, frozen concentrate, unsweetened, undiluted, canned	¾ cup	293.7
Grapefruit juice, white, frozen concentrate, undiluted	¾ cup	248.0

Food	Amount	Vit. C (mg)
Peppers, sweet, red, cooked	1 cup	232.6
Peppers, sweet, red, raw	1	190.3
Guava, raw	½ cup	188
Papayas, raw	1	187.9
Cranberry juice cocktail, bottled	1 cup	107.0
Broccoli, cooked, boiled, drained	1 cup	101.2
Strawberries, raw	1 cup	97.6
Brussels sprouts, cooked, boiled	1 cup	96.7
Orange juice, chilled	1 cup	81.9
Broccoli, raw	1 cup	78.5
Peas, edible-podded, boiled	1 cup	76.6
Kiwi fruit	1 medium	70.5
Oranges, raw, all varieties	1 medium	70
Sweet potato, canned	1 cup	67.3

Source: U.S. Department of Agriculture, Agricultural Research Service. 2008. USDA National Nutrient Database for Standard Reference, Release 21. Nutrient Data Laboratory Home Page, www.ars.usda.gov/ba/bhnrc/ndl.

◀ SEE ALSO 4.8, "Daily Vitamin Recommendations" ▶

Deficiencies and Excesses

Too little vitamin C can cause you to have bloody, swollen gums; bruise easily; or have wounds that don't heal properly. A deficiency causes **scurvy** with symptoms such as **anemia,** soft bloody gums, and (in childhood) musculoskeletal problems. People who don't consume enough vitamin C can also have dry, rough skin and experience infections more often.

Certain conditions can increase the body's need for vitamin C. These include

▶ Use of oral contraceptives and other drugs

▶ Injury

▶ Growth (during childhood and pregnancy)

▶ Smoking

▶ Illness that causes fever and infection

Too much vitamin C can cause diarrhea and gastrointestinal discomfort and increase the risk of kidney stones. Taking vitamin C supplements can interfere with tests for blood sugar level; this can be a concern for those with insulin resistance, diabetes, metabolic syndrome, or other medical conditions.

◁ *SEE ALSO Chapter 8, "Eat to Beat Disease"* ▷

◁ *SEE ALSO 10.5, "Dietary Supplements"* ▷

WORDS TO GO . . . WORDS TO GO . . . WORDS TO GO

Scurvy is a disease caused by a lack of vitamin C in the diet.

Anemia is a condition in which red blood cells or hemoglobin (proteins that carry oxygen in the body) are lower than normal.

4.7   B VITAMINS

Thiamin

Riboflavin

Niacin

Pantothenic Acid

Biotin

Vitamin B6

Folate

Vitamin B12

B vitamins, also known as B-Complex, include eight water-soluble vitamins commonly found in foods. In this subchapter, you learn the functions and food sources of each. You also learn symptoms of deficiencies for each; only some have noted symptoms for excess intakes.

Thiamin

Thiamin's functions, food sources, and potential consequences associated with deficiencies and excesses are described in the following sections.

Functions

Thiamin, also known as vitamin B1, helps all cells of the body create energy from carbohydrates. It also plays an important role in the functioning of the nervous system.

Dietary Sources

Thiamin is found in a variety of foods. Here are good or excellent food sources of thiamin:

FOOD SOURCES THAT PROVIDE AT LEAST 10 PERCENT OF THE DAILY VALUE (1.5 MILLIGRAMS) OF THIAMIN (LISTED IN DESCENDING ORDER)

Food	Amount	Thiamin (mg)
Ready-to-eat cereals	1 cup	1.500
Rice, white, long-grain, parboiled, enriched	1 cup	1.289
All-purpose white flour	1 cup	1.222

continues

FOOD SOURCES THAT PROVIDE AT LEAST 10 PERCENT OF THE DAILY VALUE (1.5 MILLIGRAMS) OF THIAMIN (LISTED IN DESCENDING ORDER) (CONTINUED)

Food	Amount	Thiamin (mg)
Pork, loin	3 oz.	1.057
Pork, cured, ham	3 oz.	0.817
Orange juice, frozen, concentrate	¾ cup	0.596
Bagels, plain, enriched	4 inch	0.535
Soybeans, edamame, boiled	1 cup	0.468
Fish, salmon, sockeye, cooked	5½ oz.	0.333
Beans, pinto, mature seeds, cooked	1 cup	0.330
Pretzels, hard, plain	10	0.304
Lima beans, cooked	1 cup	0.303
Grapefruit juice, frozen concentrate	¾ cup	0.300
Artichokes, raw	1 cup	0.300
Couscous, dry	1 cup	0.282
English muffin, plain	1	0.281
Fish, trout, rainbow, cooked	3 oz.	0.201
Nuts, macadamia, dry roasted	10–12	0.201
Corn, sweet, yellow, cooked	1 ear	0.166
Potato, baked	1	0.164
Tomato products, canned, paste	1 cup	0.157
Oranges, raw	1 medium	0.157
Beef, variety meats and byproducts, liver, cooked	3 oz.	0.150

Source: U.S. Department of Agriculture, Agricultural Research Service. 2008. USDA National Nutrient Database for Standard Reference, Release 21. Nutrient Data Laboratory Home Page, www.ars.usda.gov/ba/bhnrc/ndl.

◀ SEE ALSO 4.8, *"Daily Vitamin Recommendations"* ▶

Deficiencies and Excesses

Alcoholics might be deficient in thiamin and experience side effects including fatigue, weak muscles, and nerve damage. People being treated with hemodialysis or peritoneal dialysis and those with malabsorption syndrome need extra thiamin.

Excess thiamin is secreted in the urine and does not appear to pose a risk for adverse effects.

Riboflavin

Riboflavin's functions, food sources, and potential consequences associated with deficiencies and excesses are described in the following sections.

Functions

Riboflavin, also known as vitamin B2, is a water-soluble vitamin that helps all body cells create energy. It also helps convert tryptophan—an essential amino acid—into niacin, another B vitamin.

◄ *SEE ALSO 3.2, "Amino Acids"* ▶

4.7

Dietary Sources

Riboflavin is found in a wide variety of foods. Here are good or excellent sources in the diet:

FOOD SOURCES THAT PROVIDE AT LEAST 10 PERCENT OF THE DAILY VALUE (1.7 MILLIGRAMS) OF RIBOFLAVIN (LISTED IN DESCENDING ORDER)

Food	Amount	Riboflavin (mg)
Beef, variety meats and byproducts, liver, cooked	3 oz.	2.911
Ready-to-eat cereals	1 cup	1.710
Chicken, broilers, fryers, cooked	1 cup	1.525
Milk, canned, condensed, sweetened	1 cup	1.273
Milk, canned, evaporated	1 cup	0.796
Enriched wheat flour	1 cup	0.701
Soybeans, mature, cooked	1 cup	0.490
Yogurt, plain, low-fat	1 cup	0.486
Mushrooms, cooked	1 cup	0.468
Milk, reduced fat, 2% milkfat	1 cup	0.451
Milk, whole, 3.25% milkfat	1 cup	0.447
Cheese, cottage	1 cup	0.447
Tomato products, canned, paste	1 cup	0.401
Spinach, frozen, cooked	1 cup	0.334

continues

FOOD SOURCES THAT PROVIDE AT LEAST 10 PERCENT OF THE DAILY VALUE (1.7 MILLIGRAMS) OF RIBOFLAVIN (LISTED IN DESCENDING ORDER) (CONTINUED)

Food	Amount	Riboflavin (mg)
Nuts, almonds	24 nuts	0.287
Egg, whole, cooked	1 large	0.267
Fish, salmon, sockeye, cooked	5½ oz.	0.265
Plums, dried (prunes), stewed	1 cup	0.248

Source: U.S. Department of Agriculture, Agricultural Research Service. 2008. USDA National Nutrient Database for Standard Reference, Release 21. Nutrient Data Laboratory Home Page, www.ars.usda.gov/ ba/bhnrc/ndl.

◀ SEE ALSO 4.8, *"Daily Vitamin Recommendations"* ▶

Deficiencies and Excesses

Getting too little dietary riboflavin can cause dry, flaky, or cracked skin (especially around the nose, lips, and tongue) and eye problems including cataracts.

There are no known adverse effects from consuming too much riboflavin.

Niacin

Niacin's functions, food sources, and potential consequences associated with deficiencies and excesses are described in the following sections.

Functions

Niacin, also known as vitamin B3, is a water-soluble vitamin that helps the body create energy from carbohydrates and fatty acids. It also helps enzymes (proteins that speed up chemical reactions) function in the body.

Dietary Sources

Although some niacin can be created in the body from tryptophan, most niacin is obtained through a varied diet. Here are several good and excellent food sources of niacin:

FOOD SOURCES THAT PROVIDE AT LEAST 10 PERCENT OF THE DAILY VALUE (10 MILLIGRAMS) OF NIACIN (LISTED IN DESCENDING ORDER)

Food	Amount	Niacin (mg)
Ready-to-eat cereals	1 cup	20.010
Beef, variety meats and byproducts, liver, cooked	3 oz.	14.854

Food	Amount	Niacin (mg)
Chicken breast	4 oz. (about ½ a breast)	14.732
Fish, swordfish, cooked	3 oz.	12.497
Fish, halibut, fillet	6 oz.	11.326
Fish, tuna, light, canned in water	3 oz.	11.288
Wheat flour, white	1 cup	10.349
Fish, salmon, sockeye, cooked, fillet	5.5 oz.	10.339
Sauce, pasta, marinara	1 cup	9.793
Rice, white, long-grain, enriched	1 cup	9.503
Barley, pearled, raw	1 cup	9.208
Chicken, canned	5 oz.	8.987
Veal, leg (top round)	3 oz.	8.976
Tomato products, canned, paste	1 cup	8.059
Rice, white, long-grain	1 cup	7.755
Pork, fresh, loin, center	3 oz.	7.212
Beef, top sirloin	3 oz.	7.157
Mushrooms, cooked	1 cup	6.958
Fish, haddock, cooked	5 oz.	6.948
Couscous, dry	1 cup	6.038
Lamb	3 oz.	6.035
Chicken, broilers or fryers	3 oz.	5.939
Veal, rib, cooked	3 oz.	5.933
Turkey, all classes	3 oz.	5.744
Fish, salmon	3 oz.	5.670
Turkey roast	3 oz.	5.333
Beef, round	3 oz.	5.244
Ground turkey, cooked	1 patty (3 oz.)	3.952
Peanuts	28	3.919
Pork, cured, ham	3 oz.	3.792
Tomato products, canned, puree	1 cup	3.665
Barley, pearled, cooked	1 cup	3.239
Coffee, brewed	¼ cup	3.124

Source: U.S. Department of Agriculture, Agricultural Research Service. 2008. USDA National Nutrient Database for Standard Reference, Release 21. Nutrient Data Laboratory Home Page, www.ars.usda.gov/ba/bhnrc/ndl.

4.7

Deficiencies and Excesses

Too little niacin can cause symptoms such as diarrhea, mental disorientation, and skin problems. Those being treated with hemodialysis or peritoneal dialysis or those with malabsorption syndrome might need extra niacin.

Too much niacin (in the form of nicotinic acid, the form usually found in supplements) can cause flushed skin, liver damage, stomach ulcers, and high blood sugar.

◀ *SEE ALSO 10.5, "Dietary Supplements"* ▶

Pantothenic Acid

Pantothenic acid's functions, food sources, and potential consequences associated with deficiencies or excesses are described in the following sections.

Functions

Pantothenic acid is a water-soluble vitamin that helps create energy from carbohydrates, fats, and proteins. It also helps form hormones—messengers that deliver information from one place in the body to another.

Dietary Sources

Pantothenic acid is found in most foods. Here are some good or excellent sources in the diet:

FOOD SOURCES THAT PROVIDE AT LEAST 10 PERCENT OF THE DAILY VALUE (10 MILLIGRAMS) OF PANTOTHENIC ACID (LISTED IN DESCENDING ORDER)

Food	Amount	Pantothenic Acid (mg)
Ready to eat cereals	1 cup	10.080
Beef, variety meats and byproducts, liver, cooked	3 oz.	5.902
Mushrooms, shiitake, cooked	1 cup	5.211
Mushrooms, cooked	1 cup	3.370
Duck, domesticated, meat only, cooked	8 oz.	3.315
Milk, canned, condensed	1 cup	2.295
Seeds, sunflower seed kernels	¼ cup	2.253
Couscous, dry	1 cup	2.150
Rice, white, long-grain, parboiled, enriched, dry	1 cup	2.096

Food	Amount	Pantothenic Acid (mg)
Egg substitute, liquid	¼ cup	1.694
Yogurt, plain	1 cup	1.455
Corn, sweet, yellow, canned	1 cup	1.418
Oat bran, raw	1 cup	1.404
Peas, edible-podded, cooked	1 cup	1.371
Sweet potato, canned	1 cup	1.334
Turkey, meat only, cooked	1	1.320
Chicken, liver, cooked	1	1.307
Lentils, mature seeds, cooked	1 cup	1.263
Wheat flour, whole-grain	1 cup	1.210
Orange juice, frozen concentrate, canned	¾ cup	1.193
Cheese, cottage	1 cup	1.170
Fish, trout, rainbow, cooked	3 oz.	1.114
Fish, salmon, cooked	5½ oz.	1.085
Chicken, broilers or fryers, dark meat, meat only, cooked	3 oz.	1.059
Pumpkin, canned	1 cup	0.980
Soymilk, unfortified	1 cup	0.914
Sweet potato, cooked, boiled, without skin	5½ oz.	0.906
Milk, whole, 3.25% milkfat	1 cup	0.883
Yogurt, plain	1 cup	0.883
Egg, whole, raw, fresh	1 extra large	0.834
Cucumber, with peel, raw	1 large	0.780
Fish, salmon, smoked	3 oz.	0.740
Fish, tuna, cooked	3 oz.	0.735

4.7

Source: U.S. Department of Agriculture, Agricultural Research Service. 2008. USDA National Nutrient Database for Standard Reference, Release 21. Nutrient Data Laboratory Home Page, www.ars.usda.gov/ba/bhnrc/ndl.

◀ SEE ALSO 4.8, *"Daily Vitamin Recommendations"* ▶

Deficiencies and Excesses

A pantothenic acid deficiency is uncommon because it's found in adequate amounts in so many foods; if it does occur, symptoms can include fatigue, nausea, abdominal cramps, or difficulty sleeping.

Excessive pantothenic acid does not appear to cause any adverse or toxic symptoms or effects.

Biotin

Biotin's functions, food sources, and potential consequences associated with deficiencies or excesses are described in the following sections.

Functions

Biotin is a water-soluble vitamin that helps release energy from carbohydrates, proteins, and fats. It also helps create fatty acids and DNA.

Dietary Sources

The biotin content for many foods is unknown. However, it is found in a variety of foods, especially peanuts, almonds, egg yolks, milk, cheese, and vegetables.

Deficiencies and Excesses

Although a biotin deficiency is uncommon, some people might be at increased risk. Raw egg whites contain avidin, a protein that binds to biotin and could prevent its absorption. (Those who consume a lot of raw eggs are also at risk for foodborne illness caused by Salmonella.) People who take certain anti-seizure medications can also be at risk for a biotin deficiency. Symptoms can include hair loss; dry, scaly skin; fatigue; loss of appetite; and muscle pains. It can also contribute to delayed growth and development and convulsions and other neurological problems.

Excessive biotin intake does not appear to cause any negative health effects.

◀ *SEE ALSO 4.8, "Daily Vitamin Recommendations"* ▶

◀ *SEE ALSO 12.1, "Foodborne Pathogens"* ▶

Vitamin B6

Vitamin B6's functions, food sources, and potential consequences associated with deficiencies or excesses are described in the following sections.

Functions

Vitamin B6 (in various forms, including pyridoxine, pyridoxal, and pyridoxamine) helps the body metabolize and absorb proteins, use fats, break down glycogen (stored glucose), and create red blood cells. It also helps convert tryptophan (an essential amino acid) into niacin, another B vitamin.

Dietary Sources

Vitamin B6 is found naturally in organ meats, starchy vegetables, and noncitrus fruits as well as in some fortified foods. Here are several good or excellent food sources of vitamin B6:

FOOD SOURCES THAT PROVIDE AT LEAST 10 PERCENT OF THE DAILY VALUE (2 MILLIGRAMS) OF VITAMIN B6 (LISTED IN DESCENDING ORDER)

Food	Amount	Vitamin B6 (mg)
Ready-to-eat cereals	1 cup	2.00
Beef, variety meats and byproducts, liver	3 oz.	0.87
Rice, white, long-grain, parboiled	1 cup	0.84
Potatoes, hashed brown	1 cup	0.74
Chestnuts	1 cup	0.71
Buckwheat flour	1 cup	0..70
Fish, halibut	6 oz.	0.63
Potato, baked	1	0.63
Chicken, broilers or fryers, breast	5 oz.	0.60
Pork, fresh, loin	3 oz.	0.60
Tomato products, canned, paste	1 cup	0. 57
Bananas	1 medium	0.55
Plums, dried (prunes)	1 cup	0.54
Plantains	1 medium	0.54
Barley, pearled, raw	1 cup	0.52
Fish, haddock	5 oz.	0.52
Carrot juice, canned	1 cup	0.51
Sweet potato, canned	1 cup	0.49
Beef, top sirloin	3 oz.	0.48
Bulgur, dry	1 cup	0.48
Brussels sprouts, frozen	1 cup	0.45
Spinach, cooked	1 cup	0.44
Peppers, red, raw	1 cup	0.43
Oatmeal, instant, fortified	1 packet	0.43
Soybeans	1 cup	0.40
Beans, pinto, mature seeds, cooked	1 cup	0.39
Nuts, pistachio nuts, dry roasted	47 nuts	0.36

4.7

Source: U.S. Department of Agriculture, Agricultural Research Service. 2008. USDA National Nutrient Database for Standard Reference, Release 21. Nutrient Data Laboratory Home Page, www.ars.usda.gov/ba/bhnrc/ndl.

◀ SEE ALSO 10.3, "Functional Foods" ▶

Deficiencies and Excesses

Vitamin B6 deficiencies are rare. People who are alcoholic or have a damaged liver because of cirrhosis or hepatitis can be at risk for a vitamin B6 deficiency. Symptoms can include anemia, dermatitis and other skin problems, and neurological problems such as depression or confusion.

High intakes of supplemental B6 (2,000 mg or more per day) can lead to permanent nerve damage that causes numbness in the extremities and difficulty walking.

◀ SEE ALSO 4.8, "Daily Vitamin Recommendations" ▶

◀ SEE ALSO 10.5, "Dietary Supplements" ▶

Folate

Folate's functions, food sources, and potential consequences associated with deficiencies or excesses are described in the following sections.

Functions

Folate is a water-soluble vitamin that plays several key roles in the body. It helps

- ▶ Form red blood cells
- ▶ Metabolize proteins
- ▶ In cell growth and division
- ▶ Lower blood **homocysteine** levels (that can reduce heart disease risk)

◀ SEE ALSO 8.1, "Cardiovascular Disease" ▶

- ▶ Prevent birth defects that can occur in the spine or brain (neural tube defects such as spina bifida and anencephaly)

Dietary Sources

Folate is found naturally in a variety of foods, especially dark leafy vegetables, legumes (beans and peas), and orange juice. It is also found in fortified foods such as enriched cereals and grains. Foods naturally contain folate, whereas fortified foods and supplements contain folic acid—a more stable and better-absorbed form of folate.

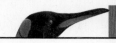

Foods are measured in dietary folate equivalents (DFEs). This unit of measure takes into account the fact that the folate found naturally in foods is less absorbed or less available to the body than folic acid. 1 DFE equals 1 microgram.

The following table shows good or excellent food sources of folate:

FOOD SOURCES THAT PROVIDE AT LEAST 10 PERCENT OF THE DAILY VALUE (400 MICROGRAMS) OF FOLATE (LISTED IN DESCENDING ORDER)

Food	Amount	Folate (mcg)
Rice, white, long-grain, enriched	1 cup	797
Ready-to-eat cereals, fortified	1 cup	716
Turkey, all classes	1 cup	486
Cornmeal	1 cup	476
Wheat flour, white	1 cup	395
Lentils, cooked	1 cup	358
Cowpeas (blackeyes, crowder, southern)	1 cup	358
Orange juice, frozen concentrate, canned	¾ cup	330
Beans, pinto, mature seeds, cooked	1 cup	294
Chickpeas (garbanzo beans, bengal gram), cooked	1 cup	282
Okra, frozen, cooked	1 cup	269
Spinach, cooked	1 cup	263
Black beans	1 cup	256
Navy beans	1 cup	255
Asparagus, frozen, cooked	1 cup	243
Bagels, plain, enriched	4 inch	201
Soybeans, edamame	1 cup	200
Collards, cooked	1 cup	177
Snacks, pretzels	10	172
Turnip greens, cooked	1 cup	170
Broccoli, cooked	1 cup	168
Brussels sprouts, frozen, cooked	1 cup	157
Lettuce, iceberg	1 head	156
Noodles, egg, enriched	1 cup	150
Artichokes	1 cup	150
Beets, cooked	1 cup	136
Papayas	1	116

continues

4.7

**FOOD SOURCES THAT PROVIDE AT LEAST 10 PERCENT
OF THE DAILY VALUE (400 MICROGRAMS) OF FOLATE
(LISTED IN DESCENDING ORDER)** (CONTINUED)

Food	Amount	Folate (mcg)
Corn, sweet, yellow, canned, cream style	1 cup	115
Chicken, liver	1	113
Sunflower seed kernels, dry roasted	¼ cup	76

Source: U.S. Department of Agriculture, Agricultural Research Service. 2008. USDA National Nutrient Database for Standard Reference, Release 21. Nutrient Data Laboratory Home Page, www.ars.usda.gov/ba/bhnrc/ndl.

◀ SEE ALSO 4.8, *"Daily Vitamin Recommendations"* ▶

Deficiencies and Excesses

A lack of folate in the diet can raise homocysteine levels (that can increase heart disease risk). It can also impair DNA synthesis; this can lead to **megaloblastic anemia** with symptoms such as weakness, fatigue, depression, irritability, forgetfulness, and disturbed sleep. Impaired DNA synthesis can also lead to diarrhea and impaired immune function. Too little folate in early pregnancy can cause an unborn fetus to develop neural tube defects such as spina bifida or anencephaly.

People are at greater risk for a folate deficiency if they are poor or suffer from eating disorders or alcoholism. Higher folate needs because of pregnancy or lactation or because of certain conditions (blood disorders or leukemia) can also make it a challenge to meet daily folate needs. Alcoholism or taking certain prescription medications can also lower folate absorption and increase deficiency risk.

Too much folate can cover up a deficiency of vitamin B12 by preventing the formation of altered red blood cells, an indicator that you're not getting enough vitamin B12. Too much folate can also make symptoms of vitamin B12 deficiency worse.

Some people might get hives or suffer from respiratory distress when they consume excess amounts of folic acid from supplements.

◀ SEE ALSO 10.3, *"Functional Foods"* ▶

Vitamin B12

Vitamin B12's functions, food sources, and potential consequences associated with deficiencies or excesses are described in the following sections.

Functions

Vitamin B12 (also called cobalamin) is a water-soluble vitamin that helps metabolize folate, another B vitamin, and build DNA and red blood cells. It also protects nerve fibers that help maintain the nervous system.

Dietary Sources

Vitamin B12 is found naturally in animal foods including meats, fish, and dairy products. Some cereals are also fortified with vitamin B12. A few plant foods naturally contain vitamin B12, but it's in a form the body cannot use.

The following table lists good or excellent food sources of vitamin B12:

FOOD SOURCES THAT PROVIDE AT LEAST 10 PERCENT OF THE DAILY VALUE (6 MICROGRAMS) OF VITAMIN B12 (LISTED IN DESCENDING ORDER)

Food	Amount	Vitamin B12 (mcg)
Clams	3 oz.	84.06
Beef, variety meats and byproducts, liver	3 oz.	70.66
Oysters	6 medium	16.35
Crab, Alaska king	3 oz.	9.78
Salmon	5½ oz.	8.99
Sardines	3 oz.	7.60
Ready-to-eat cereals, fortified	1 cup	6.00
Trout	3 oz.	4.22
Herring	3 oz.	3.63
Pollock	3 oz.	3.57
Chicken, liver	1	3.30
Lamb, shank and sirloin	3 oz.	2.24
Cheese, cottage, low-fat	1 cup	1.42
Beef, round, eye of round	3 oz.	1.39
Turkey roast, boneless	3 oz.	1.29
Yogurt, plain, low fat	1 cup	1.27
Cheese, cottage	1 cup	1.20

**FOOD SOURCES THAT PROVIDE AT LEAST 10 PERCENT
OF THE DAILY VALUE (6 MICROGRAMS) OF VITAMIN B12
(LISTED IN DESCENDING ORDER)** (CONTINUED)

Food	Amount	Vitamin B12 (mcg)
Milk, reduced fat, 2% milkfat	1 cup	1.12
Milk, whole, 3.25%	1 cup	1.07
Bologna, beef and pork	2 slices	1.03
Cheese, Swiss	1 oz.	0.95
Cheese, ricotta	1 cup	0.84
Egg, whole, extra large	1	0.75
Cheese, mozzarella	1 oz.	0.65

Source: U.S. Department of Agriculture, Agricultural Research Service. 2008. USDA National Nutrient Database for Standard Reference, Release 21. Nutrient Data Laboratory Home Page, www.ars.usda.gov/ba/bhnrc/ndl.

◀ SEE ALSO 4.8, *"Daily Vitamin Recommendations"* ▶

Deficiencies and Excesses

Too little vitamin B12 is often caused by impaired absorption. A vitamin B12 deficiency can lead to symptoms such as megaloblastic anemia that can cause serious symptoms such as brain abnormalities and breakdown of the spinal cord. Neurological symptoms include tingling or numbness of the extremities and cognitive changes such as memory loss, disorientation, and dementia. **Pernicious anemia** is also caused by a vitamin B12 deficiency. It can lead to irreversible nerve damage and possibly death.

People at risk for a vitamin B12 deficiency include

- ▶ Those with gastrointestinal problems
- ▶ Those over age 50 who absorb about 10–30 percent less vitamin B12 than they did when they were younger
- ▶ People who consume vegetarian or vegan diets and don't eat meat or dairy products
- ▶ Breastfed infants of vegan mothers

Too much vitamin B12 from foods or supplements does not appear to be harmful.

◀ SEE ALSO 10.3, *"Functional Foods"* ▶

◀ SEE ALSO 10.5, *"Dietary Supplements"* ▶

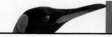

Homocysteine is an amino acid precursor of cysteine (a nonessential amino acid) and a risk factor for heart disease.

Megaloblastic anemia occurs when excess amounts of megaloblasts (large, immature red blood cells that are created when precursors fail to divide properly because of altered DNA synthesis) are created; this can be caused by a folate or vitamin B12 deficiency.

Pernicious anemia is a form of anemia caused by an autoimmune disorder that damages the lining of the stomach and inhibits the absorption of vitamin B12, leading to a deficiency.

4.7

4.8 DAILY VITAMIN RECOMMENDATIONS

Dietary reference intakes (DRIs) are established for all vitamins and include the following:

- ▶ Estimated average requirements (EARs)
- ▶ Recommended dietary allowances (RDAs)
- ▶ Adequate intakes (AIs)
- ▶ Tolerable upper intake levels (ULs)

Here are the DRIs for vitamins (note that they are expressed as RDAs or AIs):

DIETARY REFERENCE INTAKES: RECOMMENDED INTAKES FOR INDIVIDUALS FOR VITAMINS

Age Group	Vit. A mcg	Vit. C mg	Vit. D mcg	Vit. E mg	Vit. K mcg	Thiamin mg	Riboflavin mg
Infants							
0–6 months	400*	40*	5*	4*	2.0*	0.2*	0.3*
7–12 months	500*	50*	5*	5*	2.5*	0.3*	0.4*
Children							
1–3 years	300	15	5*	6	30*	0.5	0.5
4–8 years	400	25	5*	7	55*	0.6	0.6
Males							
9–13 years	600	45	5*	11	60*	0.9	0.9
14–18 years	900	75	5*	15	75*	1.2	1.3
19–50 years	900	90	5*	15	120*	1.2	1.3
51–70 years	900	90	10*	15	120*	1.2	1.3
>70 years	900	90	15*	15	120*	1.2	1.3
Females							
9–13 years	600	45	5*	11	60*	0.9	0.9
14–18 years	700	65	5*	15	75*	1.0	1.0
19–50 years	700	75	5*	15	90*	1.1	1.1
51–70 years	700	75	10*	15	90*	1.1	1.1
>70 years	700	75	15*	15	90*	1.1	1.1
Pregnancy							
14–18 years	750	80	5*	15	75*	1.4	1.4
19–50 years	770	85	5*	15	90*	1.4	1.4
Lactation							
14–18 years	1200	115	5*	19	75*	1.4	1.6
19–50 years	1300	120	5*	19	90*	1.4	1.6

Age Group	Niacin mg	Vit. B6 mg	Folate mcg	Vit. B12 mcg	Pant. Acid mg	Biotin mcg	Choline mg
Infants							
0–6 months	2*	0.1*	65*	0.4*	1.7*	5*	125*
7–12 months	4*	0.3*	80*	0.5*	1.8*	6*	150*
Children							
1–3 years	6	0.5	150	0.9	2*	8*	200*
4–8 years	8	0.6	200	1.2	3*	12*	250*
Males							
9–13 years	12	1.0	300	1.8	4*	20*	375*
14–18 years	16	1.3	400	2.4	5*	25*	550*
19–50 years	16	1.3	400	2.4	5*	30*	550*
51–70 years	16	1.7	400	2.4	5*	30*	550*
>70 years	16	1.7	400	2.4	5*	30*	550*
Females							
9–13 years	12	1.0	300	1.8	4*	20*	375*
14–18 years	14	1.2	400	2.4	5*	25*	400*
19–50 years	14	1.3	400	2.4	5*	30*	425*
51–70 years	14	1.5	400	2.4	5*	30*	425*
>70 years	14	1.5	400	2.4	5*	30*	425*
Pregnancy							
14–18 years	18	1.9	600	2.6	6*	30*	450*
19–50 years	18	1.9	600	2.6	6*	30*	450*
Lactation							
14–18 years	17	2.0	500	2.8	7*	35*	550*
19–50 years	17	2.0	500	2.8	7*	35*	550*

4.8

Recommended Dietary Allowances (RDAs) are in bold; meets the needs of 97 to 98 percent individuals in a group.

*Adequate Intakes (AI); no RDA has been established, but the amount established is somewhat less firmly believed to be adequate for individuals in a group.

Source: Institute of Medicine. Dietary Reference Intakes: The Essential Guide to Nutrient Requirements. *Washington, D.C.: National Academies Press, 2006.*

Tolerable upper intake levels are part of the DRIs. Here are the ULs that have been established for several vitamins:

DIETARY REFERENCE INTAKES: TOLERABLE UPPER INTAKE LEVELS FOR VITAMINS

Age Group	Vit. A[a] mcg	Vit. C mg	Vit. D mcg	Vit. E[bc] mg	Vit. K mcg	Thiamin mg	Riboflavin mg
Infants							
0–6 months	600	ND	25	ND	ND	ND	ND
7–12 months	600	ND	25	ND	ND	ND	ND
Children							
1–3 years	600	400	50	200	ND	ND	ND
4–8 years	900	650	50	300	ND	ND	ND
Males, Females							
9–13 years	1700	1200	50	600	ND	ND	ND
14–18 years	2800	1800	50	800	ND	ND	ND
19–70 years	3000	2000	50	1000	ND	ND	ND
>70 years	900	2000	50	1000	ND	ND	ND
Pregnancy							
14–18 years	2800	1800	50	800	ND	ND	ND
19–50 years	3000	2000	50	1000	ND	ND	ND
Lactation							
14–18 years	2800	1800	50	800	ND	ND	ND
19–50 years	3000	2000	50	1000	ND	ND	ND

Age Group	Niacin[c] mg	Vit. B6 mg	Folate[c] mcg	Vit. B12 mcg	Pant. Acid mg	Biotin mcg	Choline mg
Infants							
0–6 months	ND	ND	ND	ND	ND	ND	ND
7–12 months	ND	ND	ND	ND	ND	ND	ND
Children							
1–3 years	10	30	300	ND	ND	ND	1.0
4–8 years	15	40	400	ND	ND	ND	1.0
Males, Females							
9–13 years	20	60	600	ND	ND	ND	2.0
14–18 years	30	80	800	ND	ND	ND	3.0
19–70 years	35	100	1000	ND	ND	ND	3.5
>70 years	35	100	1000	ND	ND	ND	3.5
Pregnancy							
14–18 years	30	80	800	ND	ND	ND	3.0
19–50 years	35	100	1000	ND	ND	ND	3.5

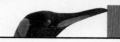

Age Group	Niacin[c] mg	Vit. B6 mg	Folate[c] mcg	Vit. B12 mcg	Pant. Acid mg	Biotin mcg	Choline mg
Lactation							
14–18 years	30	80	800	ND	ND	ND	3.0
19–50 years	35	100	1000	ND	ND	ND	3.5

ND = not determinable.

[a]*As preformed vitamin A only.*

[b]*As alpha-tocopherol or any form of supplemental alpha-tocopherol.*

[c]*Upper limits for vitamin E, niacin, and folate apply to the synthetic forms obtained from supplements, fortified foods, or a combination of the two.*

Source: Institute of Medicine. Dietary Reference Intakes: The Essential Guide to Nutrient Requirements. *Washington, D.C.: National Academies Press, 2006.*

4.8

WORDS TO GO . . . WORDS TO GO . . . WORDS TO GO

Tolerable upper intake levels (UL) are the highest amounts of a nutrient believed to be safe for most healthy people when consumed consistently. When people exceed ULs, negative health effects can occur; the more consumed, the worse the potential effects.

5

MINERALS

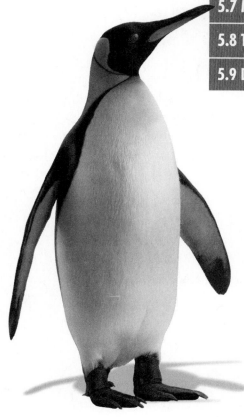

5.1 FUNCTIONS OF MINERALS

Overview

Classes

In this subchapter, you learn why minerals are so important in the body. You also learn about the three classes of minerals found in the diet and in the body.

Overview

Minerals are micronutrients that have vital functions in the body. Although they're needed in very small amounts and don't provide calories or energy the way carbohydrates, fats, and proteins do, they help the body function efficiently. Some work with enzymes, hormones, and other body proteins to support growth; others have structural roles. Unlike carbohydrates, fats, and proteins that are broken down or changed in some way after they enter the body, minerals stay intact.

◀ *SEE ALSO 1.1, "Functions of Carbohydrates"* ▶

◀ *SEE ALSO 2.1, "Functions of Fats"* ▶

◀ *SEE ALSO 3.1, "Functions of Proteins"* ▶

Unlike most vitamins, minerals can be stored by the body for long periods of time; they can also withstand light, heat, or other variables that usually degrade vitamins. Mineral absorption can, however, be affected by several food components including fiber, **phytates, oxalates,** or **polyphenols.** How acidic a person's intestinal environment is, his age, and his need and intake of the particular mineral also affect mineral absorption.

◀ *SEE ALSO 5.5, "Calcium"* ▶

Classes

Minerals are categorized by how much is needed in the diet and found in the body—not by how important they are. So even though you can need a very small amount of a particular mineral, it can still be an extremely important dietary component in the body and diet.

Major

Major minerals are needed by and stored in the body in the largest amounts. You need at least 100 milligrams of the following major minerals each day:

▶ Sodium

▶ Potassium

▶ Chloride

▶ Calcium

▶ Phosphorus

▶ Magnesium

Trace

Trace minerals are needed and stored in smaller amounts than the major minerals. You need less than 100 milligrams of the following trace minerals each day:

▶ Iron

▶ Zinc

▶ Selenium

▶ Iodine

▶ Copper

▶ Manganese

▶ Fluoride

▶ Chromium

▶ Molybdenum

Ultratrace

Ultratrace minerals are found in the body in extremely small amounts. These include

▶ Boron

▶ Nickel

▶ Silicon

▶ Arsenic

▶ Vanadium

5.1

Although daily intake recommendations for ultratrace minerals have not yet been established, and their specific functions are not fully understood, consuming a varied plant-based diet will likely provide you with adequate amounts.

WORDS TO GO . . . WORDS TO GO . . . WORDS TO GO

Phytates are acids found in plant foods as their main storage form of phosphorus; they cannot be digested by the human body.

Oxalates (also known as oxalic acids) are found in some green, leafy vegetables (such as spinach); they attach to calcium to create compounds that cannot be absorbed by the human body.

Polyphenols are chemicals found naturally in plant foods; they act as antioxidants to protect body cells against damage caused by free radicals (unstable substances found in the body and in the environment) that can contribute to the development of disease.

5.2 SODIUM

Functions

Dietary Sources

Deficiencies and Excesses

In this subchapter, you learn the key functions of sodium and where it's found in the diet. Potential problems associated with deficiencies or excesses of sodium are also described.

Functions

Sodium is a major mineral our bodies depend on to function optimally. It works with two other minerals—potassium and chloride—to maintain water balance and regulate blood pressure. Sodium also helps maintain acid/base balance, carry carbon dioxide, transmit nerve impulses, and contract muscles.

◀ *SEE ALSO 5.3, "Potassium"* ▶

Dietary Sources

About 75 percent of the sodium we consume each day comes from packaged, processed foods and beverages and restaurant foods (including fast food). Only about 25 percent comes from table salt (sodium chloride) that's added while preparing, cooking, or eating food and from sodium found naturally in foods and beverages such as eggs, fish and shellfish, meats, poultry, milk and milk products, and softened water. One teaspoon of table salt contains 2,325 mg of sodium, more than the 2,300 mg upper limit (UL), the tolerable upper intake level per day set by the Food and Nutrition Board of the National Academy of Sciences.

◀ *SEE ALSO 5.9, "Daily Mineral Recommendations"* ▶

Salt is made of sodium and chloride. Because 40% of salt is sodium, you can figure out how much salt a product contains by multiplying the milligrams of sodium listed on the Nutrition Facts Panel by 2.5. For example, if a can of soup contains 500 milligrams of sodium, 500 multiplied by 2.5 equals 1,250 milligrams of salt.

◀ *SEE ALSO 5.4, "Chloride"* ▶

Here are some commonly consumed foods and beverages that are high in sodium, which are listed in descending order:

HIGH-SODIUM FOODS AND BEVERAGES

Food	Amount	Sodium (mg)
Soup, onion, dry, mix	1 packet	3,132
Miso soup	1 cup	2,563
Bread crumbs	1 cup	2,111
All-purpose white flour, enriched	1 cup	1,588
Sauerkraut, canned	1 cup	1,560
Potato salad	1 cup	1,323
Cheeseburger	1	1,314
Tomato products, canned, sauce	1 cup	1,284
Refried beans, canned	1 cup	1,131
Pork, cured, ham, roasted	3 oz.	1,128
Beans, baked, canned	1 cup	1,114
Beans, canned with pork and tomato sauce	1 cup	1,106
Potatoes, au gratin, dry mix	1 cup	1,076
Soup, cream of chicken, canned	1 cup	1,047
Sauce, pasta, spaghetti/marinara	1 cup	1,025
Soup, beef broth or bouillon, powder, dry	1 packet	1,019
Hotdog, with corn flour coating (corndog)	1	973
Beef stew, canned entrée	1 cup	947
Cheese, cottage, low-fat, 1% milkfat	1 cup	918
Crab, Alaska king, cooked	3 oz.	911
Soy sauce	1 tbsp.	902
Soup, clam chowder, New England, canned	1 cup	888
Chicken pot pie, frozen entrée	1 small	825
Tuna salad	1 cup	824
Soup, cream of mushroom, canned	1 cup	823
Salami, cooked, beef and pork	2 slices	822
Snacks, pretzels, hard, salted	10 (2 oz.)	814
Fish, herring, Atlantic, pickled	3 oz.	740
Ham, sliced, regular	2 slices	739
Corn, sweet, yellow, canned	1 cup	730
Chickpeas, canned	1 cup	718
Cowpeas, canned	1 cup	718

continues

5.2

HIGH-SODIUM FOODS AND BEVERAGES (CONTINUED)

Food	Amount	Sodium (mg)
Sauce, teriyaki, ready-to-serve	1 tbsp.	690
Mushrooms, canned	1 cup	663
Crustaceans, shrimp	3 oz.	661
Vegetable juice cocktail, canned	1 cup	653
Frankfurter, beef and pork	1	504
Croutons, seasoned	1 cup	495
Bread, cornbread, dry mix, prepared	1 piece	467
Snacks, beef jerky, chopped and formed	1 large	438
Scallops, cooked	6 large	432
Sardines	3 oz.	430
Croissants, butter	1 (2 oz.)	424
Cheese, pasteurized, process, American	1 oz.	422
Bologna, beef and pork	2 slices	417
Cheese, blue	1 oz.	395

Source: U.S. Department of Agriculture, Agricultural Research Service. 2008. USDA National Nutrient Database for Standard Reference, Release 21. Nutrient Data Laboratory Home Page, www.ars.usda.gov/ba/bhnrc/ndl.

◀ SEE ALSO 5.9, "Daily Mineral Recommendations" ▶

Deficiencies and Excesses

Consuming less than 500 milligrams of sodium each day can cause headache, nausea, dizziness, fatigue, muscle cramps, and fainting.

Consuming too much sodium can contribute to the development of a number of health problems, including **hypertension (high blood pressure),** in those who are salt-sensitive. High blood pressure raises your risk of heart disease, stroke, heart failure, and kidney disease. Experts believe that about half of those with hypertension and about one in four who have so-called normal blood pressure can be salt-sensitive. Salt sensitivity also increases conditions such as left ventricular hypertrophy in which the heart's main pumping chamber is enlarged and does not function properly. It also raises the risk of kidney problems. Researchers believe that the following people are more likely to be salt-sensitive than their counterparts:

▶ People with hypertension, diabetes, or kidney disease

▶ People who have a family member with hypertension

▶ Middle-aged and older adults

▶ African Americans

◁ *SEE ALSO Chapter 8, "Eat to Beat Disease"* ▶

Genetic factors can also play a role in how salt intake affects blood pressure. Unfortunately, there are currently no tests you can take to determine if you're salt sensitive.

A high sodium intake can also have other harmful effects. If you consume too much sodium and at the same time don't get enough dietary calcium, the excess sodium can promote calcium loss from bones, resulting in bone fractures and osteoporosis.

◁ *SEE ALSO 5.5, "Calcium"* ▶

◁ *SEE ALSO 8.6, "Osteoporosis"* ▶

5.2

Too much sodium without enough water can also promote dehydration, which is a concern for athletes in particular. Although the kidneys of healthy people can usually excrete excessive sodium from the body, those with impaired kidney function who overconsume sodium might not be able to and instead, can store excess sodium. That can lead to edema, or swelling in the face, legs, and feet.

WORDS TO GO . . . WORDS TO GO . . . WORDS TO GO

Hypertension (high blood pressure) is persistently elevated blood pressure greater than 140/90 mmHg (millimeters of mercury).

5.3 POTASSIUM

Functions

Dietary Sources

Deficiencies and Excesses

In this subchapter, you learn the functions and dietary sources of potassium. Potential problems associated with deficiencies or excesses of potassium are also described.

Functions

Potassium is a major mineral that's involved in a variety of important processes in the body. It helps two other minerals—sodium and chloride—balance water levels, help the heart beat steadily, send nerve impulses, and support muscle contraction. Potassium can also lessen the potential effects a high-sodium diet has on blood pressure.

◄ *SEE ALSO 5.2, "Sodium"* ►

◄ *SEE ALSO 5.4, "Chloride"* ►

◄ *SEE ALSO 8.2, "Hypertension"* ►

Dietary Sources

Potassium is found in a variety of foods, such as fresh vegetables and fruits, meats, and milk products. Processed foods tend to be low in potassium (and high in sodium). Here's a list of foods and beverages that are good or excellent sources of dietary potassium, listed in descending order:

FOODS THAT CONTAIN AT LEAST 10 PERCENT
OF THE DAILY VALUE (3,500 MILLIGRAMS) OF POTASSIUM

Food	Amount	Potassium (mg)
Tomato products, canned, paste	1 cup	2,657
Orange juice, frozen concentrate, canned	¾ cup	1,436
Beet greens, cooked	1 cup	1,309
Beans, white, canned	1 cup	1,189
Dates	1 cup	1,168

Food	Amount	Potassium (mg)
Milk, canned, condensed	1 cup	1,135
Tomato products, canned, puréed	1 cup	1,098
Raisins, seedless	1 cup	1,086
Potato, baked, with skin	1 (7 oz.)	1,081
Grapefruit juice, white, frozen concentrate, canned	¾ cup	1,002
Snacks, trail mix, tropical	1 cup	993
Soybeans, green, cooked	1 cup	970
Fish, halibut, cooked	5½ oz.	916
Plantains, raw	1 medium	893
Milk, canned, evaporated, nonfat	1 cup	850
Refried beans, canned	1 cup	847
Nuts, chestnuts	1 cup	847
Spinach, cooked	1 cup	839
Tomato products, canned, sauce	1 cup	811
Plums, dried (prunes)	1 cup	796
Sweet potatoes, canned	1 cup	796
Papayas, raw	1	781
Beans, pinto, cooked	1 cup	746
Spinach, canned	1 cup	740
Prune juice, canned	1 cup	707
Sweet potato, cooked, baked in skin	1 (5 oz.)	694
Carrot juice, canned	1 cup	689
Beans, kidney, red, canned	1 cup	655
Cabbage, Chinese (bok choy), cooked	1 cup	631
Haddock, cooked, fillet	5 oz.	599
Salmon, sockeye, cooked	5 oz.	581
Yogurt, plain	1 cup	579
Parsnips, cooked	1 cup	573
Pumpkin, cooked	1 cup	564
Barley, pearled, raw	1 cup	560
Duck, domesticated, meat only, cooked	8 oz.	557
Tomato juice, canned	1 cup	556
Mushrooms, cooked	1 cup	555
Rutabagas, cooked	1 cup	554

continues

5.3

**FOODS THAT CONTAIN AT LEAST 10 PERCENT OF THE DAILY VALUE
(3,500 MILLIGRAMS) OF POTASSIUM** (CONTINUED)

Food	Amount	Potassium (mg)
Bananas, raw	1 cup	537
Clams, canned	3 oz.	534

Source: U.S. Department of Agriculture, Agricultural Research Service. 2008. USDA National Nutrient Database for Standard Reference, Release 21. Nutrient Data Laboratory Home Page, www.ars.usda.gov/ba/bhnrc/ndl.

◀ SEE ALSO 5.9, *"Daily Mineral Recommendations"* ▶

Deficiencies and Excesses

Too little dietary potassium can disrupt the balance of acids and bases in the body and contribute to bone loss and kidney stones. It can also increase the risk of hypertension. A potassium deficiency can lead to muscle cramps or weakness, confusion, and a reduced appetite. In addition, if blood levels of potassium drop too quickly, heart rhythms can be disrupted and be fatal.

People at risk for a potassium deficiency include those who consume poor diets because of alcoholism or eating disorders. Chronic diarrhea, prolonged vomiting, overuse of **diuretics** or **laxatives,** and exercise or heavy labor in hot weather that leads to high loss of body water can also cause low blood levels of potassium. People who consume a lot of black natural licorice (not artificial licorice, which is what most licorice made in the United States is), which contains a compound called glycorrhizic acid, can also excrete more potassium and have lower blood levels.

Because the kidneys typically remove excess potassium from the body, consuming too much from the diet is rarely a problem. But extremely high intakes of potassium that raise potassium blood levels too high can lead to cardiac arrest and even death. Those at risk for high blood levels of potassium include people with kidney problems and anyone taking potassium supplements. Although there is no UL for potassium intake, do not take potassium supplements without consulting your doctor first.

◀ SEE ALSO 10.5, *"Dietary Supplements"* ▶

WORDS TO GO . . .WORDS TO GO . . .WORDS TO GO

Diuretics are drugs that cause urination or water loss from the body.
Laxatives are drugs that cause looser stools or increased bowel movements.

5.4 CHLORIDE

Functions

Dietary Sources

Deficiencies and Excesses

In this subchapter, you learn the functions and dietary sources of chloride. Potential problems associated with deficiencies or excesses of chloride are also described.

Functions

Chloride is a major mineral that works with two other minerals—sodium and potassium—to regulate water balance in the body. It is also a key component of **hydrochloric acid** (or gastric juices). Chloride also helps create nerve impulses and supports immune function.

◄ *SEE ALSO 5.2, "Sodium"* ▶

◄ *SEE ALSO 5.3, "Potassium"* ▶

5.4

Dietary Sources

Most of the chloride we consume comes from sodium chloride, or table salt. Sea salt, seaweed, rye, tomatoes, lettuce, celery, olives, soy sauce, and many processed foods also contain chloride. Chloride is also found as potassium chloride in a variety of salt substitutes. Although there's limited data on the amount of chloride in various foods, you can estimate your total chloride intake by multiplying your intake of sodium in milligrams by 1.5, because table salt is 60 percent chloride. For example, if your daily sodium intake is roughly 2,500 milligrams, here's your estimated chloride intake:

2,500 milligrams sodium multiplied by 1.5 equals 3,750 milligrams of chloride.

◄ *SEE ALSO 5.9, "Daily Mineral Recommendations"* ▶

◄ *SEE ALSO 10.4, "Fat Replacers and Sugar Substitutes"* ▶

Deficiencies and Excesses

If your body loses too much fluid, from excessive sweating, vomiting (from eating disorders or other causes), diarrhea, or the use or overuse of diuretics, you can develop a chloride deficiency. If you become dehydrated, you can also be at risk for **metabolic acidosis,** a potentially fatal condition.

◀ *SEE ALSO 5.2, "Sodium"* ▶

Too much chloride from food or supplements does not appear to be toxic.

◀ *SEE ALSO 10.5, "Dietary Supplements"* ▶

WORDS TO GO . . .WORDS TO GO . . .WORDS TO GO

Hydrochloric acid is made of hydrogen and chloride that is created by gastric glands and secreted into the stomach to help the body digest and absorb nutrients.

Metabolic acidosis is a condition in which the body's acid/base balance is disturbed and blood pH levels rise (and the blood becomes more acidic).

5.5 CALCIUM

Functions

Dietary Sources

Deficiencies and Excesses

In this subchapter, you learn the functions and dietary sources of calcium. Potential problems associated with deficiencies or excesses of calcium are also described.

Functions

Calcium is a major mineral that plays several important roles in the body. It's more abundant in the body than any other mineral: most of it in bones and teeth and a very small amount in the blood and soft tissues.

Here are some of calcium's key functions:

▶ Helps form and maintain strong bones and teeth (with vitamin D and phosphorus)

▶ Helps muscles contract

▶ Helps blood vessels relax and constrict

▶ Transmits nerve impulses

▶ Helps blood clot

▶ Supports the functions of proteins (including enzymes and hormones)

▶ Helps regulate blood pressure

◀ *SEE ALSO 3.1, "Functions of Proteins"* ▶

Dietary Sources

Although calcium is found in high amounts in a variety of foods including dairy products, fish with bones, and leafy green vegetables, the amount you absorb depends on several factors. Absorption is higher when you consume less and when your needs are higher (as in infancy and pregnancy). Absorption is lower when your vitamin D intake is low. Substances such as phytates (found in nuts, seeds, and grains) or oxalates (found in spinach) can also lower your absorption of calcium, as can consuming too much wheat bran. Women might absorb less calcium after menopause because of low estrogen levels. High intakes of supplemental phosphorus or magnesium can also inhibit the absorption of calcium from foods.

◀ SEE ALSO 4.3, *"Vitamin D"* ▶

◀ SEE ALSO 10.5, *"Dietary Supplements"* ▶

Calcium is found naturally in a variety of foods. The most absorbable calcium is found in dairy foods such as milk, yogurt, and cheese. Other good or excellent sources of highly absorbable calcium are canned fish with bones; vegetables such as kohlrabi, Brussels sprouts, kale, and broccoli; and tofu and soy milk made with calcium.

Calcium is also added to some foods and beverages like orange juice, ready-to-eat cereals, breads, and yogurt products. The amount of calcium that can be absorbed from such products varies considerably.

◀ SEE ALSO 10.3, *"Functional Foods"* ▶

The following are good or excellent dietary sources of calcium:

FOODS THAT PROVIDE AT LEAST 10 PERCENT OF THE DAILY VALUE (1,000 MILLIGRAMS) OF CALCIUM (LISTED IN DESCENDING ORDER)

Food	Amount	Calcium (mg)
Milk, canned, condensed	1 cup	869
Milk, canned, evaporated, nonfat	1 cup	742
Cheese, ricotta, part skim	1 cup	669
Yogurt, plain	1 cup	452
All-purpose white flour, enriched	1 cup	423
Collards, cooked	1 cup	357
Rhubarb, cooked	1 cup	348
Sardines with bones, canned	3 oz.	325
Milk, nonfat/skim	1 cup	306
Spinach, cooked	1 cup	291
Milk, low-fat, 1% milkfat	1 cup	290
Milk, reduced-fat, 2% milkfat	1 cup	285
Milk, whole, 3.25% milkfat	1 cup	276
Soybeans, cooked	1 cup	261
Turnip greens, cooked	1 cup	249

Food	Amount	Calcium (mg)
Cheese, pasteurized, Swiss	1 oz.	219
Cheese, provolone	1 oz.	214
Cowpeas (Blackeyes), cooked	1 cup	211
Cheese, mozzarella, part skim	1 oz.	207
Cheese, cottage	1 cup	206
Cheese, cheddar	1 oz.	204
Beans, white, canned	1 cup	191
Salmon, pink, canned, solid with bone	3 oz.	181
Kale, cooked	1 cup	179
Okra, cooked	1 cup	177
Tofu, firm	¼ block (3 oz.)	163
Cabbage, Chinese (bok choy), cooked	1 cup	158
Crab, blue, canned	1 cup	136
Beans, navy, cooked	1 cup	126
Shrimp, canned	3 oz.	123
Oatmeal, instant	1 packet	110
Yogurt, frozen	½ cup	106
English muffins, plain, enriched	1	102
Rice, white, long-grain, dry, enriched	1 cup	102
Lettuce, iceberg	1 head	97
Tomato products, canned, paste	1 cup	94

5.5

Source: U.S. Department of Agriculture, Agricultural Research Service. 2008. USDA National Nutrient Database for Standard Reference, Release 21. Nutrient Data Laboratory Home Page, www.ars.usda.gov/ba/bhnrc/ndl.

◄ SEE ALSO 5.9, *"Daily Mineral Recommendations"* ►

Deficiencies and Excesses

Too little dietary calcium can contribute to bone or tooth loss and muscle cramps. Chronic low intakes can lead to osteoporosis and increase the risk of high blood pressure, colon cancer, and **preeclampsia** during pregnancy.

◄ SEE ALSO 8.2, *"Hypertension"* ►

◄ SEE ALSO 8.5, *"Cancer"* ►

◄ SEE ALSO 8.6, *"Osteoporosis"* ►

Those with kidney failure, **parathyroid disorders,** or vitamin D deficiency or those who use certain diuretic medications can develop **hypocalcemia** with symptoms such as muscle spasms or cramps, convulsions, and lethargy (although some symptoms can be due to their illnesses and not because of the calcium deficiency).

At risk for getting too little dietary calcium include

▶ Women after menopause who produce less estrogen (a hormone), lose more bone, and absorb less calcium from dietary sources

▶ Women of childbearing age who do not get their periods because of eating disorders and/or excessive physical activity

▶ Those with lactose intolerance or lactose maldigestion who consume few or no dairy foods

◀ *SEE ALSO 9.3, "Lactose Intolerance"* ▶

▶ Those who follow vegetarian or vegan eating patterns and consume few or no dairy products

Excess intakes of calcium, especially from supplements, can cause bloating, constipation, and kidney problems (such as kidney stones). It can also decrease your body's absorption of the minerals iron, magnesium, and zinc. Although it's rare, **hypercalcemia** can be caused by cancer, overproduction of parathyroid hormone (PTH) by the parathyroid gland, or excess vitamin D from supplements. Symptoms can include fatigue, confusion, decreased appetite, constipation, and impaired organ function.

◀ *SEE ALSO 10.5, "Dietary Supplements"* ▶

◀ *SEE ALSO 5.9, "Daily Mineral Recommendations"* ▶

WORDS TO GO . . .WORDS TO GO . . .WORDS TO GO

Preeclampsia is a condition that can occur during pregnancy; symptoms include high blood pressure and protein in the urine.

Parathyroid disorders involve parathyroid glands that rest on the thyroid gland in the neck and secrete parathyroid hormone (PTH) which balances calcium and phosphorus. Hyperparathyroidism is caused by secretion of excess PTH (and elevates blood calcium levels); hypoparathyroidism is caused by secretion of too little PTH (and lowers calcium levels and elevates phosphorus levels). **Hypocalcemia** is a condition in which blood levels of calcium are lower than normal.

Hypercalcemia is a condition in which blood levels of calcium are higher than normal.

5.6 PHOSPHORUS

Functions

Dietary Sources

Deficiencies and Excesses

In this subchapter, you learn the functions and dietary sources of phosphorus. Potential problems associated with deficiencies or excesses of phosphorus are also described.

Functions

Phosphorus is a mineral found throughout the body (but mostly in bone) that helps all body cells function optimally. It works with calcium and vitamin D to build and maintain strong bones and teeth. It also helps create energy from food, maintain acid/base balance, and deliver oxygen to various body tissues. Phosphorus is also a key component of **deoxyribonucleic acid (DNA), ribonucleic acid (RNA),** and **phospholipids,** which have important functions in the body.

◖ SEE ALSO 4.3, *"Vitamin D"* ▷

◖ SEE ALSO 5.5, *"Calcium"* ▷

Dietary Sources

Phosphorus is abundant in both animal-derived and plant foods. However, phosphorus from nuts, seeds, and grains is only about half as absorbable by the body as phosphorus from other food sources.

Here are some foods that are good or excellent dietary sources of phosphorus:

FOODS THAT PROVIDE AT LEAST 10 PERCENT OF THE DAILY VALUE (1,000 MG) OF PHOSPHORUS (LISTED IN DESCENDING ORDER)

Food	Amount	Phosphorus (mg)
Cornmeal, enriched, yellow	1 cup	860
Milk, canned, condensed	1 cup	774
Wheat flour, white, all-purpose, enriched	1 cup	744
Oat bran, raw	1 cup	690
Fish, halibut, cooked	6 oz.	453

continues

5.6

FOODS THAT PROVIDE AT LEAST 10 PERCENT OF THE DAILY VALUE (1,000 MG) OF PHOSPHORUS (LISTED IN DESCENDING ORDER) (CONTINUED)

Food	Amount	Phosphorus (mg)
Cheese, ricotta, part skim	1 cup	450
Duck, domesticated, meat only, cooked	8 oz.	449
Barley, pearled, raw	1 cup	442
Salmon, cooked	5½ oz.	428
Soybeans, cooked	1 cup	421
Bulgur, dry	1 cup	420
Chicken, broilers or fryers, giblets, cooked	1 cup	419
Sardines, drained, solids with bone	3 oz.	417
Wheat flour, whole-grain	1 cup	415
Pollock, cooked	3 oz.	410
Flour, buckwheat	1 cup	404
Seeds, sunflower seed kernels	¼ cup	370
Cheese, cottage, 2% milkfat	1 cup	368
Fish, swordfish, cooked	4 oz.	357
Lentils, cooked	1 cup	356
Yogurt, plain	1 cup	356
Crustaceans, blue crab	1 cup	351
Ready-to-eat breakfast cereals	½ cup	345
Beans, pinto, cooked	1 cup	251
Milk, skim	1 cup	247
Pork, fresh, loin	3 oz.	230
Trout, rainbow	3 oz.	226
Milk, whole	1 cup	222
Scallops	6 large	219
Cheese, Swiss, pasteurized	1 oz.	216
Chickpeas, canned	1 cup	216
Rice, brown, long-grain, cooked	1 cup	162
Chestnuts, roasted	1 cup	153
Cashew nuts	18	151
Almonds	24	137

Source: U.S. Department of Agriculture, Agricultural Research Service. 2008. USDA National Nutrient Database for Standard Reference, Release 21. Nutrient Data Laboratory Home Page, www.ars.usda.gov/ba/bhnrc/ndl.

◀ SEE ALSO 5.9, *"Daily Mineral Recommendations"* ▶

Deficiencies and Excesses

Although phosphorus deficiency is uncommon, it can develop in those who don't consume enough calories because of alcoholism, eating disorders, or other causes. Some drugs can also reduce phosphorus absorption in the body. Deficiency symptoms can include weak bones and muscles, fatigue, appetite loss, bone pain, and increased risk for infection.

Too much dietary phosphorus, especially from supplements, can cause diarrhea and upset stomach; over time, it can even damage the kidneys. Consuming a lot of high-phosphorus foods or beverages (including sodas made with phosphoric acid or processed foods made with phosphates) and too few calcium-rich foods can weaken bones.

◀ SEE ALSO 10.5, *"Dietary Supplements"* ▶

Some studies suggest that too much dietary fructose (from high-fructose corn syrup and other sources) can lead to greater excretion of phosphorus and lower levels in the body, especially if magnesium intake is also low.

◀ SEE ALSO 1.2, *"Sugars"* ▶

5.6

WORDS TO GO . . .WORDS TO GO . . .WORDS TO GO

Deoxyribonucleic acid (DNA) is a nucleic acid that carries genetic information; certain parts of DNA—genes—act as a set of instructions for creating body proteins.

Ribonucleic acid (RNA) is a nucleic acid that plays an important role in the creation of body proteins and in determining how genes (parts of DNA) are expressed in the body.

Phospholipids are substances that carry fats in the blood and bring nutrients in and out of body cells.

5.7 MAGNESIUM

Functions

Dietary Sources

Deficiencies and Excesses

In this subchapter, you learn the functions and dietary sources of magnesium. Potential problems associated with deficiencies or excesses of magnesium are also described.

Functions

Magnesium is a major mineral involved in hundreds of important chemical reactions in the body. More than half of the body's magnesium is stored in bones. It also helps create adenosine triphosphate (ATP), the main source of fuel for cells to rely on to create molecules, contract muscles, and carry substances around the body. Magnesium can also help lower blood pressure.

Dietary Sources

Magnesium is found abundantly in whole grains and beans. Green vegetables, nuts and seeds, milk, and some fish also contain magnesium. Here are some foods that are good or excellent dietary sources of magnesium:

FOOD SOURCES THAT PROVIDE AT LEAST 10 PERCENT OF THE DAILY VALUE (400 MILLIGRAMS) OF MAGNESIUM (LISTED IN DESCENDING ORDER)

Food	Amount	Magnesium (mg)
Flour, buckwheat	1 cup	301
Snacks, trail mix, regular	1 cup	235
Bulgur, dry	1 cup	230
Oat bran, raw	1 cup	221
Halibut, cooked	5½ oz.	170
Whole wheat flour	1 cup	166
Spinach, canned	1 cup	163
Barley, pearled, raw	1 cup	158
Spinach, fresh, cooked	1 cup	157
Cornmeal, whole-grain, yellow	1 cup	155
Seeds, pumpkin and squash, roasted	1 oz. (142 seeds)	151

Food	Amount	Magnesium (mg)
Soybeans, cooked	1 cup	148
Beans, white, canned	1 cup	134
Beans, black, cooked	1 cup	120
Tomato products, canned, paste	1 cup	110
Ready-to-eat breakfast cereals, fortified	½ cup	109
Brazil nuts	6–8 nuts	107
Lima beans, cooked	1 cup	101
Refried beans, canned	1 cup	96
Baking chocolate, unsweetened,	1 oz. square	93
Cowpeas, cooked	1 cup	91
Halibut, cooked	3 oz.	91
Muffins, oat bran	1	89
Rice, brown, long-grain, cooked	1 cup	84
Beans, kidney, red, cooked	1 cup	80
Grapefruit juice, white, frozen concentrate	¾ cup	79
Cashews	18	77
Dates	1 cup	77
Couscous, dry	1 cup	76
Haddock, cooked, fillet	5 oz.	75
Orange juice, frozen concentrate	¾ cup	72
Lentils, cooked	1 cup	71
Pine nuts	1 oz.	71
Peas, split, cooked	1 cup	71
Artichokes, cooked	1 cup	71
Milk, canned, evaporated, nonfat	1 cup	69
Mixed nuts, with peanuts	1 oz.	67
Plantains, raw	1 medium	66
Oats, quick, instant	1 cup	63
Soymilk, unfortified	1 cup	61
Potato, baked, flesh and skin	1 (7 oz.)	57
Pumpkin, canned	1 cup	56

Source: U.S. Department of Agriculture, Agricultural Research Service. 2008. USDA National Nutrient Database for Standard Reference, Release 21. Nutrient Data Laboratory Home Page, www.ars.usda.gov/ba/bhnrc/ndl.

◄ **SEE ALSO 5.9, "Daily Mineral Recommendations"** ►

5.7

Deficiencies and Excesses

Deficiencies in magnesium can occur if you don't consume enough magnesium-rich foods (and many Americans don't) or foods high in potassium or phosphorus. **Hypomagnesemia** can be seen in those with kidney disease, those with alcoholism, or those who take certain diuretic medications. Prolonged diarrhea can also put someone at risk for a deficiency. Symptoms of magnesium deficiency can include weakness, nausea, vomiting, loss of appetite, muscle cramps, irritability, and confusion.

◀ *SEE ALSO 5.3, "Potassium"* ▶

◀ *SEE ALSO 5.6, "Phosphorus"* ▶

Too little dietary magnesium can also play a role in the development of diabetes and colon cancer.

◀ *SEE ALSO 8.3, "Diabetes"* ▶

◀ *SEE ALSO 8.5, "Cancer"* ▶

Too much dietary magnesium, especially from supplements (including laxatives and antacids that often contain magnesium) can cause diarrhea, nausea, muscle weakness, confusion, irregular heartbeat, and low blood pressure. **Hypermagnesemia** seldom occurs in those who don't have kidney disease.

◀ *SEE ALSO 10.5, "Dietary Supplements"* ▶

WORDS TO GO . . .WORDS TO GO . . .WORDS TO GO

Hypomagnesemia is an abnormally low level of magnesium in the blood.
Hypermagnesemia is an abnormally high level of magnesium in the blood.

5.8 TRACE MINERALS

Iron

Zinc

Selenium

Copper

Manganese

Iodine

Fluoride

Chromium

Molybdenum

In this subchapter, you'll learn about the nine trace minerals needed by and stored in the body.

5.8

Iron

Here you learn about iron's functions and food sources, as well as potential problems associated with deficiencies or excesses of iron.

Functions

Iron is a trace mineral found in many parts of the body that performs many vital functions. It's a component of two proteins that carry oxygen from the lungs to the rest of the body: hemoglobin, found in the red blood cells, and myoglobin, found in muscle tissue. Iron is also a part of many enzymes, proteins that speed chemical reactions and create energy. Iron also supports brain development.

◄ *SEE ALSO 3.1, "Functions of Protein"* ▶

Dietary Sources

The two types of iron found in foods are heme iron and non-heme iron.

Heme iron is part of the hemoglobin and myoglobin found in animal tissues. Meats, poultry, and fish are the only dietary sources of well-absorbed heme iron.

Non-heme iron is found mainly in plant foods such as beans, leafy green vegetables, legumes, and iron-fortified foods such as grains; small amounts are found in eggs and dairy products. This form of iron is much less absorbed than heme iron. Fortunately, you can absorb more heme iron at meals if you also consume the following:

▶ A food or beverage rich in vitamin C

▶ Meat, poultry, or fish

◀ SEE ALSO 3.3, *"Animal Sources of Protein"* ▶

◀ SEE ALSO 4.6, *"Vitamin C"* ▶

◀ SEE ALSO 6.3, *"Fruits"* ▶

◀ SEE ALSO 6.4, *"Vegetables"* ▶

◀ SEE ALSO 6.6, *"Meat and Beans"* ▶

Several substances found in foods reduce iron absorption from foods. These include phytates, which are acids found in legumes (beans and peas), grains, and rice; polyphenols, which are found in coffee, tea, some fruits and vegetables, spices, and soy foods such as tofu; oxalates found in spinach, strawberries, chocolate, wheat bran, nuts, beets, and tea; and fiber. Too much calcium, phosphorus, or zinc from foods or supplements also lowers your non-heme iron absorption.

◀ SEE ALSO 10.5, *"Dietary Supplements"* ▶

Here are some foods that are good or excellent sources of dietary iron:

FOODS THAT PROVIDE AT LEAST 10 PERCENT OF THE DAILY VALUE (18 MILLIGRAMS) OF IRON (LISTED IN DESCENDING ORDER)

Food	Amount	Iron (mg)
Clams	3 oz.	23.77
Ready-to-eat cereal, fortified	1 cup	18.09
Oats, instant	1 packet	10.55
Chicken, broilers or fryers, cooked	1 cup	10.21
All-purpose white, enriched	1 cup	10.03
Rice, white, long-grain, enriched, dry	1 cup	9.73
Soybeans, boiled	1 cup	8.64
Beans, white, mature seeds, canned	1 cup	7.83
Tomato products, canned, paste	1 cup	7.81
Lentils, mature seeds, cooked	1 cup	6.59
Spinach, cooked	1 cup	6.43

Food	Amount	Iron (mg)
Oysters, cooked	3 oz.	5.91
Duck, domesticated, meat only, cooked, roasted	8 oz.	5.97
Bagels, plain, enriched	4-inch (3 oz.)	5.38
Beef, variety meats and byproducts, liver, cooked	3 oz.	5.24
Beans, kidney, red, cooked	1 cup	5.20
Barley, pearled, raw	1 cup	5.00
Baking chocolate, unsweetened	1 square (1 oz.)	4.93
Flour, buckwheat	1 cup	4.87
Chickpeas (garbanzo beans, bengal gram), cooked	1 cup	4.74
Whole-grain wheat flour	1 cup	4.66
Lima beans, cooked	1 cup	4.49
Beans, navy, cooked	1 cup	4.30
Seeds, pumpkin and squash seed kernels	1 oz. (142 seeds)	4.24
Refried beans, canned	1 cup	4.21
Potatoes, baked, skins	1 skin (2 oz.)	4.08
Peas, edible-podded, cooked,	1 cup	3.84
Mushrooms, cooked	1 cup	2.71
Beef, chuck, blade roast, cooked	3 oz.	2.62
Sardines canned in oil, drained solids with bone	3 oz.	2.48
Muffins, oat bran	1 (2 oz.)	2.39
Noodles, egg, cooked, enriched	1 cup	2.35
Chicken, liver, all classes, cooked	1	2.28
Sweet potato, canned	1 cup	2.27
Beef, ground, 85% lean meat	3 oz.	2.21
Lettuce, iceberg	1 head	2.21
Collards, cooked	1 cup	2.20
Potato, baked, flesh and skin	1 (7 oz.)	2.18

5.8

Source: U.S. Department of Agriculture, Agricultural Research Service. 2008. USDA National Nutrient Database for Standard Reference, Release 21. Nutrient Data Laboratory Home Page, www.ars.usda.gov/ ba/bhnrc/ndl.

◖ SEE ALSO 5.9, *"Daily Mineral Recommendations"* ▶

Deficiencies and Excesses

Getting too little iron is a worldwide problem. In the United States, young children, teenage girls, and women during their childbearing years are most at risk for an iron deficiency. If you have depleted iron stores, you can feel no symptoms. Eventually, you can develop **microcytic hypochromic anemia** and experience symptoms such as fatigue, weakness, increased sensitivity to cold temperatures, and behavioral changes. Children can become irritable, have a lower attention span, and have difficulty learning.

Too much iron can also have severe consequences, especially in children who accidentally overdose on iron-containing prescription or over-the-counter supplements. Symptoms of iron overload include nausea, vomiting, constipation, or diarrhea; in severe cases, a rapid heartbeat, dizziness, confusion, and even death can occur. A common inherited defect can cause iron overload disease in adults. A simple blood test can screen for this. When too much iron builds up in the body over time, it can lead to cirrhosis, diabetes, heart disease, and arthritis. Too much iron also reduces zinc absorption.

◄ *SEE ALSO Chapter 8, "Eat to Beat Disease"* ►

◄ *SEE ALSO 10.5, "Dietary Supplements"* ►

Zinc

Here you learn about zinc's functions and food sources, as well as potential problems associated with deficiencies or excesses of zinc.

Functions

Zinc is a trace mineral that's involved in many important reactions that occur in the body. It plays a key role in growth and sexual development and helps proteins such as enzymes and hormones perform their many functions. It also supports immune function and helps make DNA (genetic material). Zinc also plays a role in maintaining your senses of taste and smell.

Dietary Sources

Zinc is found in a variety of protein-rich foods including beef, liver, eggs, and seafood. It is also found in grains and legumes (beans and peas), but these foods contain phytates—acids that attach to zinc—and fiber that limits zinc absorption by the body. Zinc from animal sources is highly absorbed.

Here are some foods that are good or excellent sources of dietary zinc:

**FOODS THAT PROVIDE AT LEAST 10 PERCENT
OF THE DAILY VALUE (15 MILLIGRAMS) OF ZINC
(LISTED IN DESCENDING ORDER)**

Food	Amount	Zinc (mg)
Oysters, raw	6 medium	76.28
Ready-to-eat cereals	1 cup	15.30
Beef, chuck, blade roast, cooked	3 oz.	7.00
Crab, Alaska king, cooked	3 oz.	6.48
Duck, domesticated, meat only, cooked	8 oz.	5.75
Beef, ground, 85% lean meat, cooked	3 oz.	5.36
Beef, round, bottom round, cooked	3 oz.	4.67
Beef, top sirloin	3 oz.	4.64
Beef, variety meats and byproducts, liver	3 oz.	4.45
Barley, pearled, raw	1 cup	4.26
Flour, buckwheat	1 cup	3.74
Cheese, ricotta, part skim	1 cup	3.30
Beans, white, canned	1 cup	2.93
Oat bran, raw	1 cup	2.92
Milk, canned, condensed	1 cup	2.88
Chickpeas (garbanzo beans), canned	1 cup	2.54
Lentils, cooked	1 cup	2.51
Lobster, cooked	3 oz.	2.48
Crab cakes	1 (2 oz.)	2.45
Ground turkey, cooked	1 patty (3 oz.)	2.35
Yogurt, plain	1 cup	2.20
Wild rice, cooked	1 cup	2.20
Pork, cured, ham	3 oz.	2.18
Soybeans, mature, cooked	1 cup	1.98
Mushrooms, shiitake, cooked	1 cup	1.93
Rice, white, long-grain, parboiled, enriched, dry	1 cup	1.92

Source: U.S. Department of Agriculture, Agricultural Research Service. 2008. USDA National Nutrient Database for Standard Reference, Release 21. Nutrient Data Laboratory Home Page, www.ars.usda.gov/ba/bhnrc/ndl.

◄ *SEE ALSO 5.9, "Daily Mineral Recommendations"* ►

Deficiencies and Excesses

Zinc deficiency is rare, except in populations that live mainly on cereal grains that contain poorly absorbed zinc. However, those with gastrointestinal or digestive disorders or chronic diseases such as liver or kidney disease or with alcoholism can be at risk for a zinc deficiency. People who consume no meat (such as vegetarians or vegans) and pregnant or lactating women (who have higher zinc needs) are also at risk. Older infants (7–12 months old) who are exclusively breastfed also need more zinc.

Deficiency symptoms include impaired growth, poor wound healing and infection, taste changes, decreased immune function, and lethargy.

Although excess zinc is not stored in the body for long periods of time, in some people excess amounts from foods and/or supplements can dampen immune function and lead to hair loss, diarrhea, abdominal cramps, and vomiting and other gastrointestinal problems. Too much zinc can also cause a copper deficiency.

◄ *SEE ALSO 10.5, "Dietary Supplements"* ►

Selenium

In this section, you learn about selenium's functions and food sources, as well as potential problems associated with deficiencies or excesses of selenium.

Functions

Selenium is a trace mineral that works with vitamins C and E as an antioxidant to protect cells from damage caused by harmful free radicals. It also supports immune and thyroid function. Selenium can play a role in reducing the risk or growth of some cancers.

Dietary Sources

Selenium is found in a variety of foods, such as seafood, organ meats, nuts, and grains, though nothing tops the notable Brazil nut for selenium content. So much so, you should not eat more than two Brazil nuts per day. Here are some good or excellent dietary sources of selenium:

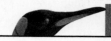

FOODS THAT PROVIDE AT LEAST 10 PERCENT
OF THE DAILY VALUE (70 MICROGRAMS) OF SELENIUM
(LISTED IN DESCENDING ORDER)

Food	Amount	Selenium (mcg)
Brazil nuts	6–8 nuts	544
Whole wheat flour	1 cup	85
Tuna salad	1 cup	85
Barley, pearled, raw	1 cup	75
Halibut, cooked, fillet	5½ oz.	74
Tuna, light, canned in water	3 oz.	68
Swordfish, cooked	4 oz.	65
Haddock, cooked, fillet	5 oz.	61
Salmon, sockeye, cooked, fillet	5½ oz.	59
White bread, enriched	1 cup	54
Mollusks, oyster, raw	6 medium	54
Herring, pickled	3 oz.	50
Duck, domesticated, meat only, cooked	8 oz.	50
Milk, canned, condensed	1 cup	45
Sardines, canned in oil with bones	3 oz.	45
Rice, white, long-grain, enriched, dry	1 cup	44
Couscous, cooked	1 cup	43
Crab, blue, canned	1 cup	43
Oat bran, raw	1 cup	43
Clams	3 oz.	41
Cheese, ricotta, part skim	1 cup	41
Pork, fresh, loin, center loin (chops)	3 oz.	41
Shrimp, canned	3 oz.	40
Noodles, egg, cooked, enriched	1 cup	38
Spaghetti, cooked, enriched	1 cup	37
Lobster, cooked	3 oz.	36
Spaghetti, whole-wheat, cooked	1 cup	36
Mushrooms, shiitake, cooked	1 cup	36
Turkey roast, boneless, roasted	3 oz.	31
Seeds, sunflower seed kernels	¼ cup	25
Beef, top sirloin, cooked	3 oz.	25
Cheese, cottage, low-fat, 2% milkfat	1 cup	22

continues

FOODS THAT PROVIDE AT LEAST 10 PERCENT OF THE DAILY VALUE (70 MICROGRAMS) OF SELENIUM (LISTED IN DESCENDING ORDER) (CONTINUED)

Food	Amount	Selenium (mcg)
Rice, brown, long-grain, cooked	1 cup	19
Egg, whole, raw, fresh, extra large	1	18

Source: U.S. Department of Agriculture, Agricultural Research Service. 2008. USDA National Nutrient Database for Standard Reference, Release 21. Nutrient Data Laboratory Home Page, www.ars.usda.gov/ba/bhnrc/ndl.

◀ SEE ALSO 5.9, *"Daily Mineral Recommendations"* ▶

Deficiencies and Excesses

Although rare, selenium deficiency can occur in those who have Crohn's disease or other severe digestive disorders or conditions or who rely on total parenteral nutrition (TPN), a method of feeding intravenously. Symptoms of a deficiency can include heart problems, hypothyroidism, and a weakened immune system. Low levels of selenium can predispose children to a rare form of heart disease and is also associated with a higher risk of cancer.

Too much selenium in the blood from foods or supplements can cause **selenosis.** Symptoms include gastrointestinal problems, hair loss, brittle nails, fatigue, irritability, and mild nerve damage.

◀ SEE ALSO 10.5, *"Dietary Supplements"* ▶

Copper

In this section, you learn about copper's functions and food sources, as well as potential problems associated with deficiencies or excesses of copper.

Functions

Copper is a trace mineral with many important functions in the body. It's part of an enzyme involved in iron metabolism and helps make red blood cells. It is also a part of enzymes that act as antioxidants to remove free radicals. Copper also helps keep the immune system, nerves, and blood vessels healthy. It also helps for the pigments in the skin, hair, and eyes.

Dietary Sources

Copper is found in a variety of foods. Here are good or excellent dietary sources of copper:

FOODS THAT PROVIDE AT LEAST 10 PERCENT
OF THE DAILY VALUE (2 MILLIGRAMS) OF COPPER
(LISTED IN DESCENDING ORDER)

Food	Amount	Copper (mg)
Beef, variety meats and byproducts, liver, cooked	3 oz.	12.40
Oysters, raw	6 medium	3.740
Lobster, cooked	3 oz.	1.649
Mushrooms, shiitake, cooked	1 cup	1.299
Candies, semisweet chocolate	1 cup	1.176
Crab, blue, canned	1 cup	1.026
Tomato products, canned, paste	1 cup	0.956
Barley, pearled, raw	1 cup	0.840
Mushrooms, cooked	1 cup	0.786
Chestnuts	1 cup	0.725
Soybeans, mature, cooked	1 cup	0.700
Cashew nuts	1 oz.	0.629
Beans, white, canned	1 cup	0.608
Sunflower seed kernels, dry roasted	¼ cup	0.586
Clams, canned	3 oz.	0.585
Chickpeas, cooked	1 cup	0.577
Duck, domesticated, meat only, cooked	8 oz.	0.511
Lentils, cooked	1 cup	0.497
Rice, white, long-grain, parboiled, enriched, dry	1 cup	0.494
Sauce, pasta, spaghetti/marinara	1 cup	0.470
Raisins, seedless	1 cup	0.461
Wheat flour, whole-grain	1 cup	0.458
Potatoes, hashed brown	1 cup	0.457
Walnuts	14 halves	0.450
Lima beans, cooked	1 cup	0.442
Couscous, dry	1 cup	0.427
Rice, white, long-grain, regular, raw, enriched	1 cup	0.407
Spinach, canned	1 cup	0.385
Beans, navy	1 cup	0.382
Pistachio nuts, dry roasted	47	0.376

continues

5.8

FOODS THAT PROVIDE AT LEAST 10 PERCENT OF THE DAILY VALUE (2 MILLIGRAMS) OF COPPER (LISTED IN DESCENDING ORDER) (CONTINUED)

Food	Amount	Copper (mg)
Mushrooms, canned	1 cup	0.367
Beans, black, cooked	1 cup	0.359
Sweet potatoes, canned	1 cup	0.354
Pecans	20 halves	0.340

Source: U.S. Department of Agriculture, Agricultural Research Service. 2008. USDA National Nutrient Database for Standard Reference, Release 21. Nutrient Data Laboratory Home Page, www.ars.usda.gov/ba/bhnrc/ndl.

Deficiencies and Excesses

Copper deficiency is rare but can occur in preterm infants and those with malabsorption conditions such as Celiac Sprue. Symptoms include anemia and bone problems.

Getting too much copper from foods or supplements can cause nausea, vomiting, or diarrhea. Too much copper can also decrease iron and zinc absorption. In rare cases, excess copper intake can cause anemia and in some cases, death.

Manganese

In this section, you learn about the functions and food sources of manganese, as well as potential problems associated with deficiencies or excesses of manganese.

Functions

Manganese is a trace mineral that has many essential functions in the body. It is a key component of many enzymes that help form cartilage, the foundation of bones and skin, and support the metabolism of amino acids (which form proteins), cholesterol, and carbohydrates.

Dietary Sources

Various plant foods and tea contain manganese. Drinking water can also supply manganese to the diet. Following are some good or excellent dietary sources of manganese.

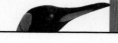

FOODS THAT PROVIDE AT LEAST 10 PERCENT OF THE DAILY VALUE (2 MILLIGRAMS) OF MANGANESE (LISTED IN DESCENDING ORDER)

Food	Amount	Manganese (mg)
Oat bran, raw	1 cup	5
Wheat flour, whole-grain	1 cup	5
Pineapple, canned, juice-packed	1 cup	3
Barley, pearled, raw	1 cup	3
Pine nuts, dried	1 oz.	2
Rice, white, long-grain, enriched, dry	1 cup	2
Spaghetti, whole-wheat, cooked	1 cup	2
Rice, brown, long-grain, cooked	1 cup	2
Okra, cooked	1 cup	2
Hazelnuts	18–20	2
Chickpeas, cooked	1 cup	2
Chestnuts, roasted	1 cup	2
Spinach, cooked	1 cup	2
Lima beans, immature seeds, cooked	1 cup	1
Soybeans, mature, cooked	1 cup	1
Pecans	20 halves	1
Collards, cooked	1 cup	1
Macadamia nuts, dry roasted	10–12	1
Lima beans, cooked	1 cup	1
Almonds	24 nuts	1

Source: U.S. Department of Agriculture, Agricultural Research Service. 2008. USDA National Nutrient Database for Standard Reference, Release 21. Nutrient Data Laboratory Home Page, www.ars.usda.gov/ ba/bhnrc/ndl.

Deficiencies and Excesses

It's uncommon to be deficient in manganese, but people with epilepsy, phenylketonuria (PKU), multiple sclerosis, and some other conditions can be deficient. Symptoms include impaired growth and bone problems.

Too much manganese from foods, water, supplements, or the environment (from dust) can be toxic. High levels can lead to irritability, hallucinations, and extreme coordination problems. People with liver problems can be especially vulnerable to the negative effects of too much manganese.

◄ *SEE ALSO 10.5, "Dietary Supplements"* ►

Iodine

In this section, you learn about iodine's functions and food sources, as well as potential problems associated with deficiencies or excesses of iodine.

Functions

Iodine is a trace mineral that is a key component of two thyroid hormones that regulate body temperature, **basal metabolic rate (BMR),** reproduction, and growth.

Dietary Sources

Iodine is found in foods in the form of iodide and iodates. Although there is limited information about specific amounts of iodine in foods, the richest sources include iodized salt and processed foods made with it, seafood, milk and dairy products, and some grains.

Deficiencies and Excesses

Deficiencies of iodine in America are uncommon because salt is iodized and we consume so much salt and salty foods. Iodine deficiency is still a risk, however, for many people around the world. People who consume a lot of raw vegetables such as cabbage, turnips, rutabagas, and cassava can be at risk because these foods contain goitrogens—compounds that prevent iodine from being absorbed and used properly. A deficiency of iodine overstimulates the thyroid gland and can cause goiter (enlarged thyroid gland) and symptoms such as intolerance to cold, weight gain, lower body temperature, and sluggishness. A severe deficiency of iodine in early pregnancy causes cretinism, characterized by stunted growth, deafness, and mental retardation.

Too much iodine especially from supplements can also cause goiter.

Fluoride

In this section, you learn about the functions and food sources of flouride, as well as potential problems associated with deficiencies or excesses of fluoride.

Functions

Flouride is a trace mineral that is essential for maintaining strong bones and teeth (especially tooth enamel) and preventing dental caries.

Sources

Few foods naturally contain fluoride; however, some is found in tea, fish (with and without bones), and canned meats and poultry. Fluoride-fortified foods and supplements (available by prescription only) and toothpaste also provide fluoride. The American Dental Association (ADA) recommends fluoride supplements for children whose drinking water supplies less than 0.6 milligrams per liter.

Deficiencies and Excesses

Too little fluoride from the diet or drinking water increases the risk of tooth decay and dental **caries.**

Too much fluoride in the diet or from toothpaste, fortified foods, and supplements can cause fluorisis (discolored teeth with specs in them). Fluoride toxicity, which can develop in those who receive hemodialysis treatments for kidney disease, can cause headaches, nausea, and abnormal heart rhythms.

Chromium

5.8

In this section, you learn about the functions and food sources of chromium, as well as potential problems associated with deficiencies or excesses of chromium.

Functions

Chromium is a trace mineral that helps the hormone **insulin** function properly to maintain normal blood glucose levels. It also helps release energy from carbohydrates and fats. Chromium can also support immune function.

Dietary Sources

There is limited information about the content of chromium in specific foods, but very small amounts are found in a variety of foods and beverages including meats and poultry, whole grains, fruits and vegetables, spices, and beer.

Deficiencies and Excesses

Too little chromium in the diet can cause high blood sugar and insulin levels. Those on TPN who have low levels can experience brain and nerve disorders.

Excessive chromium might not be a problem for most people because it's so poorly absorbed. However, animal studies suggest that chromium picolinate supplements can damage DNA—important genetic material.

◀ *SEE ALSO 10.5, "Dietary Supplements"* ▶

Molybdenum

In this section, you learn about the functions and food sources of molybdenum, as well as potential problems associated with deficiencies or excesses of molybdenum.

Functions

Molybdenum is a trace mineral needed by many enzymes in the body to help them function properly. It can support a healthy nervous system, create energy in cells, and process wastes in the kidneys.

Dietary Sources

Although little is known about how much molybdenum is found in foods, legumes (beans and peas), grains (including ready-to-eat cereals), and nuts appear to be good dietary sources.

Deficiencies and Excesses

A molybdenum deficiency does not occur in people who consume a normal diet. Those on parenteral nutrition (intravenous feedings) can develop a molybdenum deficiency and experience symptoms such as weakness, mental confusion, and night blindness.

Too much molybdenum from food or supplements can lower the body's absorption of copper, another trace mineral.

◁ *SEE ALSO 10.5, "Dietary Supplements"* ▷

WORDS TO GO . . . WORDS TO GO . . . WORDS TO GO

Microcytic hypochromic anemia is a type of anemia in which the red blood cells are smaller than normal and do not contain as much hemoglobin (a protein that carries oxygen) as normal; this can be caused by an iron deficiency or impaired production of hemoglobin.

Selenosis is a condition that can occur from excess dietary selenium intake; symptoms include hair loss, brittle nails, garlicky breath, intestinal problems, and mental changes.

Basal metabolic rate (BMR) is the amount of energy the body expends at rest; it makes up the largest portion of total calories the body expends or burns each day.

Caries is another name for cavities or tooth decay.

Insulin is a hormone naturally made by the pancreas; it helps body cells use glucose (the key fuel for the brain and nervous system) for energy by regulating blood glucose or blood sugar levels in the body.

5.9 **DAILY MINERAL RECOMMENDATIONS**

Dietary reference intakes (DRIs) are established for all minerals and include the following:

- ▶ Estimated average requirements (EARs)
- ▶ Recommended dietary allowances (RDAs)
- ▶ Adequate intakes (AIs)
- ▶ Tolerable upper intake levels (UL)

Here are the DRIs for minerals (note that they are expressed as RDAs or AIs):

DIETARY REFERENCE INTAKES (DRIS): RECOMMENDED INTAKES OF MINERALS FOR INDIVIDUALS

Age Group	Calcium mg	Chromium mcg	Copper mcg	Fluoride mg	Iodine mcg	Iron mg
Infants						
0–6 months	210*	0.2*	200*	0.01*	110*	0.27*
7–12 months	270*	5.5*	220*	0.5*	130*	11
Children						
1–3 years	500*	11*	340	0.7*	90	7
4–8 years	800*	15*	440	1*	90	10
Males						
9–13 years	1300*	25*	700	2*	120	8
14–18 years	1300*	35*	890	3*	150	11
19–30 years	1000*	35*	900	4*	150	8
31–50 years	1000*	35	900	4*	150	8
51–70 years	1200*	30*	900	4*	150	8
>70 years	1200*	30*	900	4*	150	8
Females						
9–13 years	1300*	21*	700	2*	120	8
14–18 years	1300*	24*	890	3*	150	15
19–30 years	1000*	25*	900	3*	150	18
31–50 years	1000*	25*	900	3*	150	18
51–70 years	1200*	20*	900	3*	150	8
>70 years	1200*	20*	900	3*	150	8

5.9

DIETARY REFERENCE INTAKES (DRIS): RECOMMENDED INTAKES OF MINERALS FOR INDIVIDUALS (CONTINUED)

Age Group	Calcium mg	Chromium mcg	Copper mcg	Fluoride mg	Iodine mcg	Iron mg
Pregnancy						
14–18 years	1300*	29*	1000	3*	220	27
19–30 years	1000*	30*	1000	3*	220	27
31–50 years	1000*	30*	1000	3*	220	27
Lactation						
14–18 years	1300*	44*	1300	3*	290	10
19–30 years	1000*	45*	1300	3*	290	9
19–50 years	1000*	45*	1300	3*	290	9

Age Group	Magnesium mg	Manganese mg	Molybdenum mcg	Phosphorus mcg	Selenium mcg	Zinc mg
Infants						
0-6 months	30*	0.003*	2*	100*	5*	2*
7-12 months	75*	0.6*	3*	275*	20*	3
Children						
1–3 years	80	1.2*	17	460	20	3
4–8 years	130	1.5*	22	500	30	5
Males						
9–13 years	240	1.9*	34	1250	40	8
14–18 years	410	2.2*	43	1250	55	11
19–30 years	400	2.3*	45	700	55	11
31–50 years	420	2.3*	45	700	55	11
51–70 years	420	2.3*	45	700	55	11
>70 years	420	2.3*	45	700	55	11
Females						
9–13 years	240	1.6*	34	1250	40	8
14–18 years	360	1.6*	43	1250	55	9
19–30 years	310	1.8*	45	700	55	8
31–50 years	320	1.8*	45	700	55	8
51–70 years	320	1.8*	45	700	55	8
>70 years	320	1.8*	45	700	55	8
Pregnancy						
<18 years	400	2.0*	50	1250	60	12
19–30 years	350	2.0*	50	700	60	11
31–50 years	360	2.0*	50	700	60	11

Age Group	Magnesium mg	Manganese mg	Molybdenum mcg	Phosphorus mcg	Selenium mcg	Zinc mg
Lactation						
<18 years	360	2.6*	50	1250	70	13
19–30 years	310	2.6*	50	700	70	12
31–50 years	320	2.6*	50	700	70	12

*RDA's = "**bold typed**" meets the needs of 97 to 98 percent individuals in a group.*

* = Adequate Intakes (AI) no RDI has been established, but the amount established is somewhat less firmly believed to be adequate for individuals in a group.

5.9

6

CREATING A
DAILY MEAL PLAN

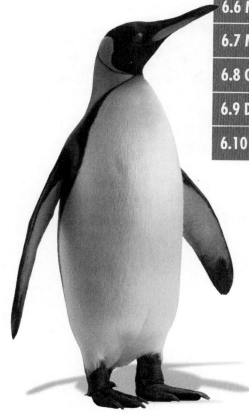

6.1 ESTIMATING YOUR DAILY CALORIE NEEDS

Estimated Energy Requirements

Estimating Your Calorie Needs

In this subchapter, you learn how to estimate the number of calories you should consume each day to achieve and maintain a healthy body weight.

Estimating Your Energy Requirements

Energy or calorie needs vary from person to person and are based on a number of factors, including age, sex, height, weight, and activity level. Here's a table you can use as a guide for determining how many calories to consume each day. The calorie levels are based on the Institute of Medicine's **estimated energy requirements (EER)** and activity levels. They're based on the calories needed to maintain energy balance in individuals who are at healthy body weights.

DAILY CALORIE LEVELS

AGE	MALES Activity level Sedentary[a]	Mod. active[b]	Active[c]	FEMALES Activity level Sedentary[a]	Mod. active[b]	Active[c]
2	1000	1000	1000	1000	1000	1000
3	1000	1400	1400	1000	1200	1400
4	1200	1400	1600	1200	1400	1400
5	1200	1400	1600	1200	1400	1600
6	1400	1600	1800	1200	1400	1600
7	1400	1600	1800	1200	1600	1800
8	1400	1600	2000	1400	1600	1800
9	1600	1800	2000	1400	1600	1800
10	1600	1800	2200	1400	1800	2000
11	1800	2000	2200	1600	1800	2000
12	1800	2200	2400	1600	2000	2200
13	2000	2200	2600	1600	2000	2200
14	2000	2400	2800	1800	2000	2400
15	2200	2600	3000	1800	2000	2400
16	2400	2800	3200	1800	2000	2400
17	2400	2800	3200	1800	2000	2400
18	2400	2800	3200	1800	2000	2400
19-20	2600	2800	3000	2000	2200	2400
21-25	2400	2800	3000	2000	2200	2400

AGE	MALES Activity level			FEMALES Activity level		
	Sedentary[a]	Mod. active[b]	Active[c]	Sedentary[a]	Mod. active[b]	Active[c]
26-30	2400	2600	3000	1800	2000	2400
31-35	2400	2600	3000	1800	2000	2200
36-40	2400	2600	2800	1800	2000	2200
41-45	2200	2600	2800	1800	2000	2200
46-50	2200	2400	2800	1800	2000	2200
51-55	2200	2400	2800	1600	1800	2200
56-60	2200	2400	2600	1600	1800	2200
61-65	2000	2400	2600	1600	1800	2000
66-70	2000	2200	2600	1600	1800	2000
71-75	2000	2200	2600	1600	1800	2000
76 & up	2000	2000	2400	1600	1800	2000

*Calorie levels are based on the Estimated Energy Requirements (EER) and activity levels from the Institute of Medicine Dietary Reference Intakes Macronutrients Report, 2002.

[a]Sedentary = less than 30 minutes a day of moderate physical activity in addition to daily activities.

[b]Mod. active = at least 30 minutes up to 60 minutes a day of moderate physical activity in addition to daily activities.

[c]Active = 60 or more minutes a day of moderate physical activity in addition to daily activities.

Source: mypyramid.gov.

6.1

◀ SEE ALSO 6.2, "Your Daily Meal Pattern" ▶

After you determine your daily calorie goals, you can determine a meal pattern that helps you meet your calorie and nutrient goals.

Estimating Your Calorie Needs

The following equation, called the Mifflin-St. Jeor equation, can also be used to estimate your **resting metabolic rate (RMR);** this can then be used along with an activity factor (a number based on how physically active you are) to estimate your daily calorie needs. The equation is based on weight, height, and age. Do the following:

1. Convert your weight in pounds to kilograms. Because there are 2.2 pounds in 1 kilogram, divide your weight in pounds by 2.2; that will tell you how many kilograms you weigh.

2. Convert your height in inches. Because 1 inch equals 2.54 centimeters, multiply your height in inches by 2.54; that will tell you how tall you are in centimeters.

3. Determine your resting metabolic rate (RMR):

▶ Women: RMR = 9.99 × weight (in kg) + 6.25 × height (in cm) − 4.92 × age − 161

▶ Men: RMR = 9.99 × weight (in kg) + 6.25 × height (in cm) − 4.92 × age + 5

4. Determine your daily physical activity level and multiply that by your RMR:

▶ If sedentary, multiply RMR by 1.25.

▶ If you have low activity (you walk at a pace of 3–4 miles per hour and walk the equivalent of about 1.5–2.9 miles per day), multiply RMR by 1.5.

▶ If active (you walk at a pace of 3–4 miles per hour and walk the equivalent of about 5.3–9.9 miles per day), multiply RMR by 1.75.

▶ If very active (you walk at a pace of about 3–4 miles per hour and walk the equivalent of 12.3–22.5 miles per day), multiply RMR by 2.2.

As an example, here's how a 40-year-old female who is 5'3" tall, weighs 145 pounds, and walks about 2 miles per day, would figure out her daily calorie needs using the following equation:

1. 145 pounds divided by 2.2 pounds per kilogram equals 65.9 kilograms.

2. 5'3" equals 63 inches (there are 12 inches per foot); 63 inches multiplied by 2.54 centimeters equals 160 centimeters.

3. 9.99 × 65.9 kg + 6.25 × 160 cm − 4.92 × 40 − 161 = 1301 (RMR).

4. 1301 (RMR) × 1.5 = 1951 kilocalories.

In this example, this woman would need approximately 1,951 calories to maintain her body weight.

WORDS TO GO . . .WORDS TO GO . . .WORDS TO GO

Estimated energy requirement (EER) is the daily requirement for energy; it is calculated from a set of equations and factors that account for an individual's energy intake, energy expenditure, age, sex, weight, height, and physical activity level.

Resting metabolic rate (RMR) is a clinical measurement of an individual's resting energy expenditure; it is determined 3–4 hours after eating or performing significant physical activity and accounts for 60%–75% of an individual's total energy expenditure. Although RMR is often used interchangeably with basal metabolic rate (BMR), RMR is often slightly higher than BMR.

6.2 YOUR DAILY MEAL PATTERN

MyPyramid Basics

Daily Food Guide

In this subchapter, you are introduced to MyPyramid, the new food pyramid based on current national dietary guidelines. You also learn what a healthful balanced dietary pattern looks like for you based on your individual daily calorie needs.

MyPyramid Basics

In 2005, MyPyramid was unveiled to replace the **Food Guide Pyramid.** MyPyramid provides Americans age 2 and above with an outline for how to eat in a more healthful way each day.

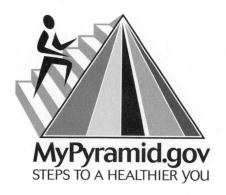

6.2

MyPyramid is based on the 2005 version of the **Dietary Guidelines for Americans.** Together, they are designed to help Americans consume an appropriate amount of calories to support a healthy body weight and, at the same time, maximize nutrient intake.

MyPyramid emphasizes three key principles:

▶ Variety—Consume items from all the basic food groups (fruits, vegetables, grains, meat and beans, milk, and oils) and subgroups (including dark green, deep orange, and starchy vegetables as well as legumes such as beans and peas).

▶ Proportion—Consume more fruits, vegetables, whole grains, and fat-free or low-fat milk or milk products and eat fewer foods rich in saturated or trans fats, added sugars, cholesterol, salt, and alcohol.

▶ Moderation—Choose foods that offer lower amounts of saturated and trans fats, added sugars, cholesterol, salt, and alcohol.

Daily Food Guide

MyPyramid provides 12 daily meal patterns to meet individual calorie needs for Americans age 2 and above. Calorie levels range from 1,000 to 3,200 calories; individual calorie recommendations are based on age, sex, and activity level.

◀ SEE ALSO 6.1, *"Estimating Your Daily Calorie Needs"* ▷

After you've determined your daily calorie needs to help you maintain your current weight or to help you achieve and maintain a healthier body weight, you can use the following table as a guide for what and how much to consume each day.

The following table includes the recommended daily intake amounts for foods and beverages from the various food categories as outlined in MyPyramid.

RECOMMENDED DAILY AMOUNTS OF FOOD FROM EACH FOOD GROUP

Food Group	Daily Calorie Level											
	1,000	1,200	1,400	1,600	1,800	2,000	2,200	2,400	2,600	2,800	3,000	3,200
Fruits (cups)	1	1	1.5	1.5	1.5	2	2	2	2	2.5	2.5	2.5
Vegetables (cups)	1	1.5	1.5	2.0	2.5	2.5	3	3	3.5	3.5	4	4
Grains: Whole (oz. eq*)	1.5	2	2.5	3	3	3	3.5	4	4.5	5	5	5
Refined (oz. eq*)	1.5	2	2.5	2	3	3	3.5	4	4.5	5	5	5
Meat and Beans (oz. eq*)	2	3	4	5	5	5.5	6	6.5	6.5	7	7	7
Milk (cups)	2	2	2	3	3	3	3	3	3	3	3	3
Oils (tsp.)	3	3.5	3.5	5	5	6	6	7	7	8	9	11
Discretionary Calories	165	171	171	132	195	267	290	362	410	426	512	648

*ounce equivalents

Source: MyPyramid, United States Department of Agriculture, 2005.

As you can see, MyPyramid breaks down foods and beverages into specific food categories. Here's what's included in each one:

- ▶ Fruits—All fresh, frozen, canned, and dried fruits and fruit juices made or prepared without added sugars or fats.

◀ *SEE ALSO 6.3, "Fruits"* ▶

- ▶ Vegetables—All fresh, frozen, and canned vegetables and vegetable juices made or prepared without added sugars or fats. Subcategories include dark green, deep orange, and starchy vegetables as well as legumes (beans and peas; these can also be counted in the Meat and Beans category).

◀ *SEE ALSO 6.4, "Vegetables"* ▶

- ▶ Grains—Whole grains and foods made with whole grains (for example, wheat, oats, cornmeal, barley, or other cereal grains) and refined grains (for example, white flour, degermed cornmeal, white bread, and white rice).

◀ *SEE ALSO 6.5, "Grains"* ▶

- ▶ Meat and Beans—Meats and poultry (lean), fish, eggs, legumes (beans and peas), tofu and other soy foods, nuts, nut butters, and seeds.

◀ *SEE ALSO 3.3, "Animal Sources of Protein"* ▶

◀ *SEE ALSO 3.4, "Plant Sources of Protein"* ▶

◀ *SEE ALSO 6.6, "Meat and Beans"* ▶

- ▶ Milk—All low-fat or fat-free milks, yogurts, frozen yogurts, dairy desserts, cheeses, and lactose-free and lactose-reduced products and made or prepared without added sugar.

◀ *SEE ALSO 6.7, "Milk"* ▶

- ▶ Oils—Vegetable oils; mayonnaise; some salad dressings; and vegetable oil spreads and soft margarines that are added to foods during processing, cooking, or at the table.

◀ *SEE ALSO 6.8, "Oils"* ▶

- ▶ Discretionary Calories—Calories from added sugars, solid fats, or alcohol, or calories from the extra fat or sugar in foods made with or that naturally contain more fat and sugar (for example, high-fat meats or fruit made with added sugar).

◀ *SEE ALSO 6.9, "Discretionary Calories"* ▶

WORDS TO GO . . .WORDS TO GO . . .WORDS TO GO

The **Food Guide Pyramid** was the nutrition guide of the United States Department of Agriculture used before the development of MyPyramid in 2005.

The **Dietary Guidelines for Americans** is a set of science-based guidelines published every 5 years by the United States Department of Health and Human Services (DHHS) and the United States Department of Agriculture (USDA). They're used to create national nutrition policies, and a new version is expected in 2010.

6.3 FRUITS

Overview

Daily Recommended Amounts

In this subchapter, you learn why it's important to include fruits in your diet.

Overview

Fruits contain several key nutrients and other beneficial substances. They provide simple carbohydrates and are naturally low in fat and sodium and contain no cholesterol. Because of their high water and fiber content, fruits tend to be filling and can therefore be useful allies if you're trying to lose or manage your weight. They're also relatively low in calories. Studies show that consuming fruits and vegetables as part of a healthful, nutritious diet can reduce the risk for cardiovascular diseases (including strokes), type 2 diabetes, and some cancers.

◀ SEE ALSO Chapter 8, "Eat to Beat Disease" ▶

Although all fruits are healthful, some are standouts. Whole fruits typically contain fewer calories and more fiber than more concentrated—and more caloric—varieties such as dried fruits or fruit juices. Some high-fiber fruits include pears, raspberries, strawberries, bananas, and guava.

◀ SEE ALSO 1.4, "Fiber" ▶

Many fruits provide good sources of vitamins and minerals. Some fruits that are high in vitamin A include mango, cantaloupe, and apricots. Vitamin C–rich fruits include guava, papaya, oranges, and orange juice. Fruits rich in potassium include bananas, plantains, and oranges.

◀ SEE ALSO 4.2, "Vitamin A" ▶

◀ SEE ALSO 4.6, Vitamin C ▶

◀ SEE ALSO 5.3, "Potassium" ▶

Some fruits are also rich sources of phytochemicals such as **carotenoids** (beta carotene, lutein, and zeaxanthin), **flavonoids** (anthocyanidins, flavanols, flavonones, and proanthocyanidins), and **phenols** (caffeic acid, ferulic acid, and resveratrol); following are a few examples.

► Carotenoids—Citrus fruits, peaches, apricots, pink grapefruit, watermelon, pumpkin, and guava

► Flavonoids—Strawberries, blueberries, raspberries, cherries, red grapes, apples, and citrus fruits

► Phenols—Apples, pears, citrus fruits, and purple grape juice

◄ SEE ALSO 10.3, *"Functional Foods"* ►

Daily Recommended Amounts

MyPyramid recommends between 1 and 2½ cups of fruit each day depending on your individual daily calorie allotment.

◄ SEE ALSO 6.1, *"Estimating Your Daily Calorie Needs"* ►

◄ SEE ALSO 6.2, *"Your Daily Meal Pattern"* ►

Each of the following counts as approximately ½ cup of fruit (or about 60 calories):

► ½ cup cut up, raw, cooked, or frozen fruit

► 1 piece of fruit (1 small orange, peach, or banana)

► ½ cup 100% fruit juice (orange juice, cranberry juice, or grape juice)

► ¼ cup dried fruit (1 small box of raisins, 1½ ounces)

WORDS TO GO . . . WORDS TO GO . . . WORDS TO GO

Carotenoids are a group of compounds naturally found in plant foods (including fruits and vegetables) that provide their deep yellow, orange, and red colors. Carotenoids convert to vitamin A in the body and can work as antioxidants, boosting immunity, promoting heart health, and supporting vision.

Flavonoids are a group of compounds found naturally in plant foods (including fruits and vegetables). They can act as antioxidants, supporting heart health, helping maintain brain function, and supporting health of the urinary tract.

Phenols are compounds found naturally in plants and plant foods. They can work as antioxidants, supporting a healthy heart, and helping maintain vision.

6.4   VEGETABLES

Overview

Daily Recommended Amounts

Weekly Recommended Amounts

6.4

After reading this subchapter, you should understand why vegetables are important dietary components and know how much to aim for each day and each week.

Overview

Vegetables are naturally low in fat and free of cholesterol. Although some contain simple carbohydrates, starchy vegetables and legumes (beans and peas) are considered complex carbohydrates.

◀ SEE ALSO Chapter 1, *"Carbohydrates"* ▶

Many vegetables are rich in vitamins and minerals including vitamin A, vitamin C, potassium, and iron. Some examples are

> ▶ Vitamin A—Sweet potatoes, carrots, spinach, collards, kale, mixed veggies, turnip greens, beet greens, winter squash, mustard greens, and red sweet peppers

◀ SEE ALSO 4.2, *"Vitamin A"* ▶

> ▶ Vitamin C—Red sweet peppers, green peppers, Brussels sprouts, kohlrabi, broccoli, sweet potatoes, tomato juice, cauliflower, and kale

◀ SEE ALSO 4.6, *"Vitamin C"* ▶

> ▶ Potassium—Sweet potatoes, tomato paste, beet greens, white potatoes, white beans, tomato products (paste, sauce, and juice), carrot juice, lima beans, lentils, kidney beans, and split peas

◀ SEE ALSO 5.3, *"Potassium"* ▶

> ▶ Iron—Soybeans, white beans, lentils, spinach, kidney beans, chickpeas, cowpeas, lima beans, soybeans, navy beans, and tomato paste

◀ SEE ALSO 5.8, *"Trace Minerals"* ▶

Vegetables also contain fiber and many are high in water content; because of this, they bulk up meals and fill you up while providing fewer calories.

◀ SEE ALSO 1.4, *"Dietary Fiber"* ▶

Vegetables also contain a variety of phytochemicals that can promote health and protect against diseases such as cancer. Here are some phytochemicals and some of the vegetables that contain them:

▶ Flavonoids—Eggplant, radishes, and red cabbage

▶ Quercetin—Onions

▶ Carotenoids—Beets

▶ Lycopene—Tomatoes, especially processed tomato products (such as canned tomato products, spaghetti sauce, and ketchup)

Cruciferous vegetables such as cauliflower, broccoli, cabbage, and kale contain glucosinolates, indoles, and other substances that can reduce the risk of some cancers.

◀ *SEE ALSO 8.5, "Cancer"* ▶

Daily Recommended Amounts

MyPyramid recommends between 1 and 4 cups (or 2 to 8 half cup servings) of vegetables each day depending on individual calorie needs.

◀ *SEE ALSO 6.1, "Estimating Your Daily Calorie Needs"* ▶

◀ *SEE ALSO 6.2, "Your Daily Meal Pattern"* ▶

In general, here's what counts as 1 cup of vegetables:

▶ 1 cup of cut-up, raw, or cooked vegetables or vegetable juice

▶ 2 cups of leafy green vegetables

Vegetables vary in their calorie contents. Most contain between 40 and 60 calories per cup. However, starchy vegetables such as corn, green peas, and white potatoes have about 140 calories per cup. It's important to be mindful of the calorie differences when you choose your vegetables and to keep portions of more caloric choices (such as starchy vegetables) small to maximize nutrients and keep calorie intake in check.

Weekly Recommended Amounts

MyPyramid suggests weekly intakes for several vegetable subcategories. Following are weekly goals for vegetable intake depending on your individual calorie needs.

WEEKLY GOALS FOR VEGETABLE INTAKE

Daily Calorie Intake	Suggested Number of Cups Based on Daily Calorie Intake			
	Dark Green	Orange	Starchy	Other
1,000	1	½	1½	3½
1,200	1½	1	2½	4½
1,400	1½	1	2½	4½
1,600	2	1½	2½	5½
1,800	3	2	3	6½
2,000	3	2	3	6½
2,200	3	2	6	7
2,400	3	2	6	7
2,600	3	2½	7	8½
2,800	3	2½	7	8½
3,000	3	2½	9	10
3,200	3	2½	9	10

Source: MyPyramid, United States Department of Agriculture, 2005.

Here are some examples of vegetables included in each subcategory:

▶ Dark green vegetables—Bok choy, broccoli, collard greens, dark green leafy lettuce, kale, mesclun, mustard greens, romaine lettuce, spinach, turnip greens, and watercress

▶ Orange vegetables—Acorn squash, butternut squash, carrots, Hubbard squash, pumpkin, and sweet potatoes

▶ Starchy vegetables—Corn, green peas, lima beans (green), and potatoes

▶ Other vegetables—Artichokes, asparagus, bean sprouts, beets, Brussels sprouts, cabbage, cauliflower, celery, cucumbers, eggplant, green beans, green or red peppers, mushrooms, okra, onions, parsnips, tomatoes, tomato juice, and vegetable juice

6.4

WORDS TO GO . . . *WORDS TO GO* . . . WORDS TO GO

Cruciferous vegetables are all members of the cabbage family of vegetables; includes kale, collard greens, broccoli, cauliflower, cabbage, Brussels sprouts, and turnips. They're loaded with phytochemicals, vitamins, minerals, and fiber.

6.5 GRAINS

Overview

Daily Recommended Amounts

After reading this subchapter, you should understand the difference between whole grains and refined grains and how they contribute to an overall healthful diet. You also learn how much of each to consume each day.

Overview

Grains are rich sources of complex carbohydrates (that supply glucose, the main fuel needed by the brain and body for energy) and contain some plant protein as well. They're also good sources of vitamins and minerals such as folate, thiamin, niacin, iron, and magnesium.

◀ SEE ALSO 3.4, *"Plant Sources of Protein"* ▶

◀ SEE ALSO 4.7, *"B Vitamins"* ▶

◀ SEE ALSO 5.7, *"Magnesium"* ▶

◀ SEE ALSO 5.8, *"Trace Minerals"* ▶

There are two types of grains: whole grains and refined grains.

Whole Grains

Whole grains are foods that include all the essential parts of the entire grain seed or kernel (including the nutrients and other components found in those parts). A whole grain includes three key components: the **bran** (outer layer), the **germ** (innermost part), and the **endosperm** (middle layer).

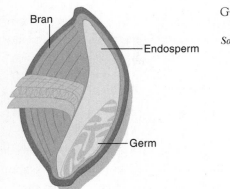

Grain anatomy.

Source: Bob's Red Mill.

Some commonly consumed whole grain foods include whole wheat bread, oatmeal, whole wheat pasta, brown rice, whole wheat crackers, and popcorn.

Whole grains are often good sources of dietary fiber (even though amounts vary from about ½ gram to 4 grams per serving). They also contain the B vitamins folate, thiamin, riboflavin, and niacin, as well as the minerals iron, magnesium, and selenium.

◀ SEE ALSO 1.4, "Dietary Fiber" ▶

◀ SEE ALSO 4.7, "B Vitamins" ▶

◀ SEE ALSO Chapter 5, "Minerals" ▶

Whole grains also contain various phytochemicals such as saponins, ferulic acid, and lignans that can help protect cells from being destroyed by free radicals and protect against chronic disease.

As part of a healthy diet, whole grains can promote gastrointestinal health, reducing constipation and the development of diverticulosis. Consuming whole grains can also reduce the risk of heart disease, stroke, type 2 diabetes, and some cancers and support a healthy immune system. Compared with refined grains, fiber-rich whole grains are more slowly digested, which keeps you feeling full for longer and can help you consume fewer calories.

6.5

Refined Grains

Refined grains are made when whole grains are milled into flour to make breads, pasta, cereals, and other foods. Unfortunately, milling removes two key components of whole grains—the bran and germ. That means the end product does not have many healthful nutrients such as fiber, vitamins, minerals, and phytochemicals that are specifically found in those parts of the whole grain. Only the endosperm, which contains some protein, vitamins, and minerals, is unaffected by milling and is intact on the final product produced.

Fortunately, many refined grains are **enriched** with several B vitamins and iron. Despite this, refined grains are usually not as nutritious as whole grains because they are missing other nutrients, especially minerals, phytochemicals, and fiber.

◀ SEE ALSO 10.3, "Functional Foods" ▶

Refined grains often have less fiber and are digested and absorbed more quickly than whole grains and therefore tend to be less filling. Many refined grains also have a high **glycemic index (GI).** Research suggests that people who consume too many high-GI foods have more than double the risk for developing diabetes compared with those who consume fewer high-GI foods. High-GI foods enter the bloodstream quickly, which raises blood sugar levels. That then triggers the pancreas to release the hormone insulin into the bloodstream, which lowers blood sugar to more normal levels. Too many, or large portions of, high-GI foods can overwork the pancreas, which keeps releasing more and more insulin. Too much insulin in the blood can contribute to high blood cholesterol, high blood triglycerides, low HDL or ("good" cholesterol), and increased blood clotting.

◄ SEE ALSO Chapter 8, "Eat to Beat Disease" ►

A recent study also found people who consumed a lot of refined carbohydrates (refined grains as well as added sugars) doubled their risk for heart disease.

◄ SEE ALSO 1.2, "Sugars" ►

◄ SEE ALSO 6.9, "Discretionary Calories" ►

Many of the starchy, baked, snack-type grains we commonly consume are made primarily or solely of refined grains. Some common refined grains include white breads; rolls; flour tortillas; white rice; pasta; crackers; and snack foods such as pretzels, potato chips, cakes, and cookies.

Daily Recommended Amounts

Here are MyPyramid's recommendations for daily intake of whole grains and refined grains depending on your individual calorie needs:

DAILY GOALS FOR GRAIN INTAKE
SUGGESTED NUMBER OF 1-OUNCE EQUIVALENT SERVINGS
BASED ON DAILY CALORIE INTAKE

Daily Calorie Intake	Whole Grains	Refined Grains
1,000	1½	1½
1,200	2	2
1,400	2½	2½
1,600	3	2½
1,800	3	3
2,000	3	3
2,200	3½	3½
2,400	4	4
2,600	4½	4½
2,800	5	5
3,000	5	5
3,200	5	5

Source: MyPyramid, United States Department of Agriculture, 2005.

A one-ounce equivalent serving of grains equals approximately:

- ► 1 cup ready-to-eat cereal flakes or puffs
- ► ½ to ¾ cup ready-to-eat cereal nuggets
- ► ½ cup cooked cereal
- ► 1 ounce dry or ½ cup cooked pasta or rice
- ► 1 slice of bread
- ► 1 ounce of crackers

WORDS TO GO . . .WORDS TO GO . . .WORDS TO GO

The **bran** is the protective multilayered outermost component of a whole-grain seed or kernel. It contains antioxidants; B vitamins; the minerals iron, zinc, copper, and magnesium; fiber; and phytochemicals.

The **germ** is the innermost part of the grain that contains unsaturated fats, some protein, several B vitamins, vitamin E, and phytochemicals.

The **endosperm** is the largest part of the whole grain seed or kernel. It contains carbohydrates (specifically starches), protein, and small amounts of vitamins and minerals.

Enriched grains contain many of the nutrients lost during processing. The B vitamins thiamin, riboflavin, and niacin and the mineral iron are added back after whole grains are milled to produce refined flour.

Glycemic index (GI) measures how much a food or beverage raises blood sugar or blood glucose levels. Foods or beverages that have higher GI values raise blood sugar more rapidly (and higher) than those with lower GI values.

6.5

6.6 MEAT AND BEANS

Overview

Daily Recommended Amounts

Weekly Recommended Amounts

In this subchapter, you learn which foods count in the Meat and Beans food category and why they're important in the diet. You also learn how much to aim for each day and, in some cases, each week.

Overview

Foods in the Meat and Beans category include meats, poultry, fish, eggs, nuts and seeds, and legumes (beans and peas). These foods provide a variety of key nutrients such as protein, B vitamins (including niacin, thiamin, riboflavin, and vitamin B6) and vitamin E and the minerals iron, zinc, and magnesium.

◀ SEE ALSO Chapter 3, "Proteins" ▶

◀ SEE ALSO Chapter 4, "Vitamins" ▶

◀ SEE ALSO Chapter 5, "Minerals" ▶

Because some foods in the Meat and Beans category, especially meat and poultry, are high in total fat, saturated fat, or cholesterol, MyPyramid urges Americans to consume these foods in lean, or low-fat forms (for example, skinless white meat chicken instead of dark meat chicken with the skin on) to minimize saturated fat and cholesterol.

◀ SEE ALSO 2.4, "Saturated Fats" ▶

◀ SEE ALSO 2.5, "Trans Fats" ▶

◀ SEE ALSO 2.6, "Dietary Cholesterol" ▶

Daily Recommended Amounts

MyPyramid recommends from two to seven one-ounce equivalent servings of Meat and Beans each day depending on your individual calorie needs.

◀ SEE ALSO 6.1, "Estimating Your Daily Calorie Needs" ▶

◀ SEE ALSO 6.2, "Your Daily Meal Pattern" ▶

The following count as a 1-ounce equivalent of meat or beans (about 55 calories):

- ▶ 1 ounce lean meat
- ▶ 1 ounce lean poultry
- ▶ 1 ounce fish
- ▶ 1 egg
- ▶ ¼ cup legumes (beans, peas, and tofu)
- ▶ ½ ounce nuts and seeds

Nuts, seeds, and nut butters also contain natural oils, which is why they count in the Oil food category as well. Here's how to count some of the nuts, seeds, and nut butters you consume in your meal plan:

- ▶ ½ ounce nuts or seeds (about 14 peanuts, 9 cashews, or 12 almonds) count as 1 Meat and Beans equivalent and 1.5 teaspoons Oil equivalent
- ▶ 1 tablespoon peanut butter counts as 1 Meat and Beans and 2 teaspoons Oil
- ▶ ½ ounce hazelnuts (about 10) counts as 1 Meat and Beans equivalent and 2 teaspoons Oil equivalent

◀ *SEE ALSO 6.2, "Your Daily Meal Pattern"* ▶

◀ *SEE ALSO 6.8, "Oils"* ▶

6.6

Because nuts, seeds, and nut butters are **energy-dense,** it's important to watch portion sizes to maximize the health benefits and stay within your recommended daily calories.

Weekly Recommended Amounts

Above and beyond its daily recommendations for the Meat and Beans category, MyPyramid makes a minimum weekly recommendation for the intake of legumes (beans and peas) to help Americans reap the many health benefits associated with their intake. Following is how many cups to aim for each day based on your individual daily calorie needs.

SUGGESTED WEEKLY AMOUNT OF LEGUMES

Daily Calorie Intake	Number of Cups
1,000	½
1,200–1,400	1
1,600	2½

continues

SUGGESTED WEEKLY AMOUNT OF LEGUMES (CONTINUED)

Daily Calorie Intake	Number of Cups
1,800–2,400	3
2,600–3,200	3½

◀ SEE ALSO 3.4, *"Plant Sources of Protein"* ▶

◀ SEE ALSO 6.1, *"Estimating Your Daily Calorie Needs"* ▶

Because legumes are energy-dense (they contain about 230 calories per cup), it's important to keep portions small so you don't overconsume calories.

WORDS TO GO . . .WORDS TO GO . . .WORDS TO GO

Energy-dense foods contain a lot of calories for a relatively small portion size.

6.7 MILK

Overview

Daily Recommended Amounts

This subchapter, you learn which foods and beverages count in the Milk food category and why they're important in the diet. You also learn how much to aim for each day.

Overview

Milk, yogurt, cheese, and other dairy foods count in the Milk food category in MyPyramid. These foods are important vehicles for high-quality protein and are excellent sources of the minerals calcium and potassium and of vitamin D (added through fortification). They also contain vitamin A, some B vitamins (including riboflavin, niacin, and vitamin B12), and the minerals phosphorus and magnesium.

◀ *SEE ALSO 3.3, "Animal Sources of Protein"* ▶

◀ *SEE ALSO Chapter 4, "Vitamins"* ▶

◀ *SEE ALSO Chapter 5, "Minerals"* ▶

6.7

There are many low-fat and nonfat milk products to choose from, but Americans consume a lot of full-fat dairy products like whole milk and cheese. Although small amounts of high-fat dairy foods can certainly fit into a healthful diet, too much can contribute too much total fat, saturated fat, and cholesterol; this can promote weight gain and increase the risk of heart disease and other health conditions.

◀ *SEE ALSO 2.4, "Saturated Fats"* ▶

◀ *SEE ALSO 2.6, "Dietary Cholesterol"* ▶

◀ *SEE ALSO 8.1, "Cardiovascular Disease"* ▶

Consuming low-fat dairy foods in place of higher-fat dairy foods can reduce your calorie, total fat, and saturated fat intake. And because of the protein they contain, dairy products can help you feel full.

Daily Recommended Intakes

MyPyramid encourages Americans aged 2 and above to consume nonfat or low-fat milk, yogurt, and cheese to maximize nutrients and minimize total fat and saturated fat intake. To fight childhood obesity and promote heart health, the American Academy of Pediatrics (AAP) recently recommended reduced-fat milk instead of whole milk for children between the ages of 12 months and 2 years who are at risk of becoming overweight or have a family history of obesity, high cholesterol, or heart disease. The AAP continues to recommend a transition to low-fat and nonfat milk and dairy products from age 2 on.

MyPyramid recommends from two to three one-cup equivalents of milk depending on your daily calorie intake.

◀ SEE ALSO 6.1, *"Estimating Your Daily Calorie Needs"* ▶

◀ SEE ALSO 6.2, *"Your Daily Meal Pattern"* ▶

With the exception of skim milk, which contains about 80 calories per cup, all other milk, yogurt, and cheese options count as Milk + Discretionary Calories.

◀ SEE ALSO 6.9, *"Discretionary Calories"* ▶

If you don't consume dairy foods because you don't like the taste, avoid all animal foods, or have **lactose intolerance,** it will be more challenging to obtain adequate calcium (not to mention other key nutrients such as vitamin D) in your diet. But turn to fortified ready-to-eat cereals, fortified orange juice, fish (such as canned sardines and pink salmon, eaten with bones), beans (including soybeans and white beans), soy foods (such as tofu or soy milk processed with calcium), and dark greens (such as spinach, kale, broccoli, and okra) since they're good nondairy sources of calcium.

◀ SEE ALSO 4.3, *"Vitamin D"* ▶

◀ SEE ALSO 5.5, *"Calcium"* ▶

◀ SEE ALSO 9.3, *"Lactose Intolerance"* ▶

WORDS TO GO . . .WORDS TO GO . . .WORDS TO GO

Lactose intolerance is a condition in which a person lacks the enzyme lactase; this enzyme is needed in the small intestine to digest lactose, the sugar found in milk and other dairy products.

6.8 OILS

Overview

Daily Recommended Amounts

In this subchapter, you learn which foods count in the Oils food category. You also learn how much to aim for in a day.

Overview

Oils are fats that are liquid at room temperature. They occur naturally in plant foods (such as nuts and seeds, avocados, and olives) and in fish. Oils contain a mixture of fats, and they are important dietary sources of **monounsaturated** and **polyunsaturated fatty acids.**

Many oils are also good sources of vitamin E. Oils from plant sources are cholesterol free.

◄ *SEE ALSO 4.4, "Vitamin E"* ▢

Although the monounsaturated and polyunsaturated fats found in vegetable oils and foods naturally rich in oils do not raise blood cholesterol levels, the oils provide a lot of calories in relatively small portions. Because we get most of the oils we need naturally from foods, we need to limit the amount of vegetable oils and other fats we add to foods while cooking or at the table.

◄ *SEE ALSO Chapter 2, "Fats"* ▢

Daily Recommended Amounts

MyPyramid recommends 3–11 teaspoons of oils per day depending on your individual calorie needs.

Each of the following are the equivalent of 1 teaspoon of oil and contain approximately 45 calories:

▶ 1 teaspoon of oil (including canola, corn, cottonseed, olive, safflower, soybean, sunflower, sesame, or walnut oils); mayonnaise; mayonnaise-type salad dressing; or margarine (soft, trans fat free)

▶ 1 tablespoon Italian or Thousand Island salad dressing; mayonnaise (light or low-fat)

▶ 2 tablespoons light salad dressing

▶ ⅓ cup avocado, sliced

▶ Olives (15 small or 10 large black pitted; 7 green [queen size]; 12 stuffed green olives)

▶ ½ oz. of most nuts (14 peanuts, 12 almonds, or 9 cashews) or 1 tablespoon nut butters (these also count as 1-oz. equivalents of Meat and Beans)

◀ *SEE ALSO 6.6, "Meat and Beans"* ▶

WORDS TO GO . . . WORDS TO GO . . . WORDS TO GO

Monounsaturated fatty acids are healthful unsaturated fats that provide calories and are liquid at room temperature but can become more solid when refrigerated.

Polyunsaturated fatty acids are essential unsaturated fats that need to be obtained by the diet because the body cannot make them; they're healthful unsaturated fats that provide the body with calories and are usually liquid at room temperature or when refrigerated.

6.9   DISCRETIONARY CALORIES

Overview

Daily Recommended Amounts

Discretionary Calories in Foods and Beverages

In this subchapter, you learn what discretionary calories are, how many are allotted for each day, and the amounts you'll find in some commonly consumed foods and beverages.

Overview

In addition to the basic food categories, MyPyramid provides a **discretionary calorie allowance**; these are extra calories that are available every day in addition to the calories provided by the lean, low-fat, and low-sugar foods and beverages in key food groups. You can use your discretionary calories for larger portions of foods, or to consume a desired fatty or sugary treat (for example, full-fat cheese instead of low-fat cheese). You can also count foods that don't fit neatly in any of the basic food categories as discretionary calories; these include solid fats (like butter or cream cheese), sugary foods, and alcoholic beverages.

Daily Recommended Amounts

MyPyramid recommends between 165 and 648 discretionary calories per day depending on your daily calorie needs.

◄ SEE ALSO 6.1, *"Estimating Your Daily Calorie Needs"* ▶

◄ SEE ALSO 6.2, *"Your Daily Meal Pattern"* ▶

Discretionary Calories in Foods and Beverages

If you use your discretionary calories to have extra portions of nutrient-dense foods and beverages, following is how they count toward your discretionary calorie allotment.

6.9

DISCRETIONARY CALORIES FOUND IN ITEMS
FROM MYPYRAMID'S FOOD CATEGORIES

Food Category	Amount of Discretionary Calories
Fruit, ½ cup	60
Vegetables:	
Dark green, deep yellow, other, ½ cup	25
Vegetables: starchy, ½ cup	70
Grains, 1-oz. equivalent	80
Meat and Beans:	
Poultry, fish, eggs, 1-oz. equivalent	55
Legumes, ½ cup	115
Nuts and seeds, ½ oz.	100
Dairy Foods:	
Skim milk, 1 cup	80
Oils, 1 teaspoon	45

Here are some foods and beverages that count toward your daily intake of discretionary calories. Many must also be counted as a portion from their respective food groups (for example, 1% milk counts as 1 cup of milk plus 20 discretionary calories). Some, like alcohol and butter, count only as discretionary calories.

DISCRETIONARY CALORIES FOUND IN ITEMS
FROM MYPYRAMID'S FOOD CATEGORIES

Food Category	Discretionary Calories
Milk	
1% milk, 1 cup	20
2% milk (reduced fat), 1 cup	40
Whole milk, 1 cup	65
Low-fat chocolate milk, 1 cup	75
Cheddar cheese, 1½ ounces	90
Whole-milk mozzarella, 1½ ounces	45
Processed cheese (American), 2 ounces	90
Plain nonfat yogurt, 1 cup	20
Plain low-fat yogurt, 1 cup	60
Fruit-flavored low-fat yogurt, 1 cup	110–115

Food Category	Discretionary Calories
Milk	
Frozen yogurt, 1 cup	140
Ice cream, vanilla, 1 cup	205
Cheese sauce, ¼ cup	75
Meat and Beans	
Regular ground beef, 80% lean, 3 oz., cooked	65
Roasted chicken thigh with skin, 3 oz.	70
Fried chicken with skin and batter, 3 wings	335
Beef sausage, precooked, 3 oz., cooked	180
Pork sausage, 3 oz., cooked	125
Beef bologna, 3 slices	100
Grains	
Blueberry muffin, 1 small, 2 oz.	45
Croissant, 1 medium, 2 oz.	95
Biscuit, plain, 1–2.5"	60
Cornbread, 1 piece, 2½ × 2½ × 1¼"	50
Graham crackers, 2 large pieces	50
Whole wheat crackers, 5	20
Round snack crackers, 7	35
Chocolate chip cookies, 2 large	70
Cake-type doughnuts, plain, 2 mini doughnuts, 1.5"	50
Glazed doughnut, yeast type, 1 medium, 3¾"	165
Cinnamon sweet roll, 3 oz.	100
Vegetables	
French fries, 1 medium order	325
Onion rings, 1 order (8–9 rings)	160
Beverages	
Regular soda, 12 oz. can	155
Regular soda, 20 oz. bottle	260
Fruit punch, 1 cup	115

6.9

continues

DISCRETIONARY CALORIES FOUND IN ITEMS
FROM MYPYRAMID'S FOOD CATEGORIES (CONTINUED)

Food Category	Discretionary Calories
Beverages	
Table wine, 5 oz.	115
Beer (regular), 12 oz.	145
Beer (light), 12 oz.	110
Distilled spirits (80 proof), 1½ oz.	95
Extras	
Butter, 1 tsp.	35
Stick margarine, 1 tsp.	35
Cream cheese, 1 tbsp.	50
Heavy (whipping) cream, 1 tbsp.	50
Dessert topping, frozen, semi-solid, 1 tbsp.	15
Gravy, canned, ¼ cup	30

Source: MyPyramid, United States Department of Agriculture, 2005.

WORDS TO GO . . . WORDS TO GO . . . WORDS TO GO

Discretionary calorie allowance is the amount of calories left in a person's total energy or calorie allowance after accounting for the number of calories needed to meet recommended nutrient intakes from low-fat, low-sugar foods and beverages.

6.10 DAILY WATER NEEDS

Overview

Daily Recommended Amounts

Water is vital to life. After reading this subchapter, you should understand the important functions of water in both the body and the diet, which foods and beverages are high in water content, and how much water to aim for each day.

Overview

Although humans can survive a few weeks without food, we can't last more than a few days without water. About 55%–75% of the human body is made of water. Water has several vital functions in the body:

▶ It carries oxygen and nutrients such as glucose and fat to muscles and helps eliminate wastes such as carbon dioxide and lactic acid from the body.

▶ It regulates body temperature.

▶ It prevents dehydration.

▶ It reduces fluid retention.

▶ It provides moisture to the skin, ears, nose, and throat.

▶ It aids digestion because it's a key component of saliva and gastric juices.

▶ It helps fiber pass through the body more easily (to prevent **constipation** or gastrointestinal discomfort).

◀ SEE ALSO 1.4, *"Dietary Fiber"* ▷

▶ It protects joints, organs (including the brain, eyes, and spinal cord), and other body tissues from shock.

About 80% of our daily water needs typically comes from water and other beverages, but about 20% comes from water-rich foods such as fruits, vegetables, grains, meats, fish, and cheese.

Daily Recommended Amounts

The Institute of Medicine recommends the following intakes of "water" (from foods and all beverages) each day:

6.10

▶ Women—11 cups of water

▶ Men—16 cups of water

Because only 20 percent of daily water needs can typically be met from foods, 80 percent should come from liquids including water. To meet these needs, women should aim for the equivalent of 9 cups of fluids and men about 13 cups of fluids.

Because daily water needs increase during pregnancy and breastfeeding, the Institute of Medicine recommends the following daily intakes:

▶ Pregnancy—13 cups of water

▶ Breastfeeding—16 cups of water

Daily "water" needs can be met by drinking any beverage including water, milk, 100 percent fruit juice, coffee, tea, and other beverages.

Water needs also increase in a variety of conditions and situations, including the following:

▶ If you exercise, especially for long periods of time or in warm weather

▶ When the weather is hot and you sweat a lot

▶ When the weather is cold and your skin is less moist

▶ If you live in or visit places in high altitudes (greater than 8,200 feet)

▶ When you travel on an airplane where air is recirculated

▶ When you have a fever, vomit, or have diarrhea

▶ If you have certain health conditions such as kidney, liver, thyroid, adrenal, or heart disease and retain more water

Because young children (including infants) don't sweat as much and don't tolerate high temperatures as well as adults, their fluid intakes need to be monitored more closely. Also, older adults are less able to sense thirst than younger adults, and may drink less water than they need and should also be monitored. The best way for most people to gauge that they're getting adequate water is to make sure they're urinating at least every 2 or 3 hours; urine should be pale yellow or clear in color, although sometimes dietary supplements or medicines can alter the color of urine to make it appear more concentrated.

WORDS TO GO . . .WORDS TO GO . . .WORDS TO GO

Constipation is a condition characterized by difficult or infrequent bowel movements.

7

WEIGHT MANAGEMENT

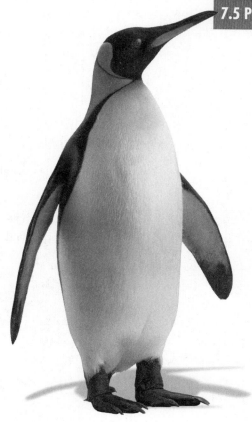

7.1 ENERGY BALANCE

Energy Intake

Energy Expenditure

In this subchapter, you learn about the two components of energy balance: energy intake and energy expenditure. Factors that influence how many calories you consume and how many you burn are discussed. Calories burned during common physical activities and exercises are provided as well.

Energy Intake

Energy intake is the amount of energy, expressed as calories, supplied by the diet. When you consume foods and beverages, calories created by the digestion of carbohydrates, fats, and proteins provide the body with energy to help it function optimally. Carbohydrates and proteins contain 4 calories per gram, and fats contain 9 calories per gram.

◀ *SEE ALSO 1.1, "Functions of Carbohydrates"* ▶

◀ *SEE ALSO 2.1, "Functions of Fats"* ▶

◀ *SEE ALSO 3.1, "Functions of Proteins"* ▶

Although alcohol is another dietary source of calories or energy for the body, it contains few key nutrients to keep us healthy. One gram of alcohol contains 7 calories.

◀ *SEE ALSO 6.9, "Discretionary Calories"* ▶

Factors That Affect Energy Intake

How many calories we consume on any given day is affected by an interaction of our genetic makeup and the environment we are exposed to early in life and our adult years. **Hunger** is a basic sensation that drives us to eat. The foods and beverages we prefer to consume are determined by genes and exposure to foods and beverages early in life. The sight and smell of foods or beverages influence our **appetite;** highly palatable and appealing foods such as sweets or fried foods can increase appetite and lead us to eat (even if we're not hungry), while the sight or smell of some foods can diminish appetite.

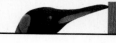

Other factors that affect our energy intake include

▶ Nutrients in food

▶ Portion sizes

▶ Psychological factors

▶ Social factors

Foods that are high in protein (for example, lean meats, poultry, fish, soy foods, nuts and seeds, and low-fat dairy foods), fiber (for example, fruits, vegetables, and whole grains), or both (for example, beans) promote **satiety,** by filling us up more than foods that are lower in protein or fiber.

◀ *SEE ALSO 1.4, "Dietary Fiber"* ▶

◀ *SEE ALSO 3.3, "Animal Sources of Protein"* ▶

◀ *SEE ALSO 3.4, "Plant Sources of Protein"* ▶

◀ *SEE ALSO Chapter 6, "Creating a Daily Meal Plan"* ▶

Portion sizes also influence how much we eat and drink. Often, we consume more when we're served larger portions than when we are presented with smaller portions. Because many people eat many of their meals away from home and foods and beverages (whether from restaurants, food carts, or vending machines, for example) are offered in bloated portion sizes, it's no surprise that many of us consume more than we intend to without even realizing it and subsequently gain weight.

7.1

◀ *SEE ALSO 7.3, "Overweight and Obesity"* ▶

Emotions such as stress or anxiety can also affect energy intake. Some people eat more when feeling down; others might shun or dramatically decrease food intake in response to negative emotions. Also, those who tend to eat more when they're stressed often turn to high-calorie, high-fat, or high-sugar but nutrient-poor "comfort foods" to make themselves feel better (even though these foods actually may do the opposite and make them feel worse, promote swings in their blood sugar levels, increase hunger, or contribute to overeating and subsequent weight gain).

Dining with others can encourage people to eat more than they would if they were alone. However, eating in front of the television or computer monitor, while listening to music, while driving, or when otherwise distracted can lead to mindless munching.

Energy Expenditure

Energy expenditure is the amount of calories the body burns or uses up each day. **Basal energy expenditure (BEE)** counts the calories used just for breathing and other basic body functions. It accounts for a surprising 75% of the total calories you burn each day. Total daily energy expenditure additionally includes the energy used to

▶ Process food (this includes digesting and absorbing food, moving nutrients around the body, and storing nutrients for later use; represents about 10% of total energy expenditure)

▶ Support physical activity and exercise (this includes all body movements; varies from person to person and depends on the type of activities you choose and how often, how intensely, and for how long you engage in physical activity or exercise)

◀ SEE ALSO 7.5, *"Physical Activity and Exercise"* ▶

Factors That Affect Energy Expenditure

Although genes largely determine whether your resting metabolic rate (RMR) is high or low, several environmental factors affect how many calories you burn each day. RMR is relatively consistent in an individual but can vary widely from person to person; this accounts for the marked differences in individual daily calorie needs.

◀ SEE ALSO 6.1, *"Estimating Your Daily Calorie Needs"* ▶

Those who have more lean body mass have a higher RMR than those with a lower proportion of lean body mass, which means they burn more calories. Men often have a higher RMR than women because they tend to weigh more and have more lean body mass. Younger people also tend to have a higher RMR than older people because getting older often causes a loss of muscle tissue and an increase in body fat. RMR might also increase during

▶ Growth (examples: pregnancy, infancy, and childhood)

▶ Cold weather (RMR increases to warm the body)

▶ Physical stress, illness, or fever

Daily calorie expenditure can also vary tremendously among individuals because of body movements not related to exercise. Nonexercise activity thermogenesis (NEAT) is the energy expended during daily activities such as sitting, standing, and fidgeting. Studies have shown that lean people expend more energy on these subtle body movements than obese people.

Calories Burned in Exercise

Although the number of calories you burn doing different activities varies depending on individual factors, here are some estimates based on different body weights:

**ESTIMATED NUMBER OF CALORIES BURNED
DURING PHYSICAL ACTIVITY BASED ON BODY WEIGHT**

Activity (one-hour duration)	Weight of person and calories burned			
	120 pounds (54 kilograms)	160 pounds (73 kilograms)	200 pounds (91 kilograms)	240 pounds (109 kilograms)
Aerobics, high impact	383	511	637	763
Aerobics, low impact	273	365	455	545
Aerobics, water	219	292	364	436
Backpacking	383	511	637	763
Basketball game	437	584	728	872
Bicycling, < 10 mph, leisure	218	292	364	436
Bowling	164	219	273	327
Canoeing	191	256	319	382
Dancing, ballroom	164	219	273	327
Football, touch, flag, general	437	584	728	872
Golfing, carrying clubs	246	329	410	491
Hiking	328	438	546	654
Ice skating	382	511	637	763
Jogging, 5 mph	437	584	728	872
Racquetball, casual, general	382	511	637	763
Rollerblading	683	913	1,138	1,363
Rope jumping	546	730	910	1,090
Rowing, stationary	382	511	637	763
Running, 8 mph	737	986	1,229	1,472

continues

7.1

ESTIMATED NUMBER OF CALORIES BURNED
DURING PHYSICAL ACTIVITY BASED ON BODY WEIGHT (CONTINUED)

Activity (one-hour duration)	Weight of person and calories burned			
	120 pounds (54 kilograms)	160 pounds (73 kilograms)	200 pounds (91 kilograms)	240 pounds (109 kilograms)
Skiing, cross-country	382	511	637	763
Skiing, downhill	273	365	455	545
Skiing, water	328	438	546	654
Softball or baseball	273	365	455	545
Stair treadmill	491	657	819	981
Swimming, laps	382	511	637	763
Tae kwon do	546	730	910	1,090
Tai chi	218	292	364	436
Tennis, singles	437	584	728	872
Volleyball	218	292	364	436
Walking, 2 mph	137	183	228	273
Walking, 3.5 mph	208	277	346	414
Weightlifting, free weight, Nautilus, or universal type	164	219	273	327

Source: Ainsworth B. E., W. L. Haskell, M. C. Whitt, M. L. Irwin, A. M. Swartz, S. J. Strath, W. L. O'Brien, D. R. Bassett Jr., K. H. Schmitz, P. O. Emplaincourt, D. R. Jacobs Jr., A. S. Leon. Compendium of Physical Activities: An Update of Activity Codes and MET Intensities. Medical Science Sports Exercise, *September 2000. 32 (9 Suppl.): S498-504.*

Hunger is a painful or unpleasant sensation in your stomach caused by the lack of food.

Appetite is a mental desire for food that might have nothing to do with hunger; it often results from pleasant sensations associated with foods or can even be triggered by the time of day or by smells.

Satiety is a feeling of fullness (satiation) that occurs after you have eaten enough; this sensation reduces the desire for more food.

Basal energy expenditure (BEE), also called resting energy expenditure (REE), is the energy or calories needed by the body to support basic physiological functions such as breathing, moving blood around the body, and building and repairing body cells. BEE accounts for most of the total energy used by the body each day and is fairly constant.

7.1

7.2 DETERMINING A HEALTHY BODY WEIGHT

Body Mass Index

Waist Circumference

In this subchapter, you learn about two common measurements used to assess body weight and where fat is distributed in the body. You also see whether your measurements put you at increased risk for diet-related diseases and conditions.

Body Mass Index

Body mass index (BMI) is a common measurement used to assess body weight; it is also an indirect but reliable way of gauging a person's body fat level.

BMI is determined from your weight and height. Here's the formula for calculating it:

▶ BMI = weight (in pounds) divided by height (in inches, squared) and multiplied by 704.5

For example, here's how a woman who weighs 130 pounds and is 5 feet 4 inches tall would determine her BMI using the formula:

1. Convert height to inches: 5 feet × 12 inches per foot = 60 inches; because the woman is 5 feet 4 inches, add 4 inches; height in inches = 64

2. Multiply answer from #1 by itself: 64 × 64 = 4096

3. Divide answer from #2 by 130: 4096 ÷ 130 = 0.0317

4. Multiply answer from #3 by 704.5 to get BMI: 0.0317 × 704.5 = 22.36 = BMI

The following table can also be used by those 20 and older to determine BMI.

After you know your BMI, you can see which of the following weight categories it falls in:

▶ Underweight—BMI below 18.5

▶ Normal weight—BMI 18.5–24.9

▶ Overweight—BMI 25.0–29.9

▶ Obese—BMI ≥ 30

▶ Extremely obese—BMI ≥ 40

BODY MASS INDEX FOR ADULTS AGED 19 AND ABOVE

To determine your BMI, find your height in the left column. Then move across the same row to the number closest to your weight. The number at the top of that column is your BMI.

BMI	19	20	21	22	23	24	25	26	27	28	29	30	31	32	33	34	35	36
Height (inches)	Body Weight (pounds)																	
58	91	96	100	105	110	115	119	124	129	134	138	143	148	153	158	162	167	172
59	94	99	104	109	114	119	124	128	133	138	143	148	153	158	163	168	173	178
60	97	102	107	112	118	123	128	133	138	143	148	153	158	163	168	174	179	184
61	100	106	111	116	122	127	132	137	143	148	153	158	164	169	174	180	185	190
62	104	109	115	120	126	131	136	142	147	153	158	164	169	175	180	186	191	196
63	107	113	118	124	130	135	141	146	152	158	163	169	175	180	186	191	197	203
64	110	116	122	128	134	140	145	151	157	163	169	174	180	186	192	197	204	209
65	114	120	126	132	138	144	150	156	162	168	174	180	186	192	198	204	210	216
66	118	124	130	136	142	148	155	161	167	173	179	186	192	198	204	210	216	223
67	121	127	134	140	146	153	159	166	172	178	185	191	198	204	211	217	223	230
68	125	131	138	144	151	158	164	171	177	184	190	197	203	210	216	223	230	236
69	128	135	142	149	155	162	169	176	182	189	196	203	209	216	223	230	236	243
70	132	139	146	153	160	167	174	181	188	195	202	209	216	222	229	236	243	250
71	136	143	150	157	165	172	179	186	193	200	208	215	222	229	236	243	250	257
72	140	147	154	162	169	177	184	191	199	206	213	221	228	235	242	250	258	265
73	144	151	159	166	174	182	189	197	204	212	219	227	235	242	250	257	265	272
74	148	155	163	171	179	186	194	202	210	218	225	233	241	249	256	264	272	280
75	152	160	168	176	184	192	200	208	216	224	232	240	248	256	264	272	279	287
76	156	164	172	180	189	197	205	213	221	230	238	246	254	263	271	279	287	295

continues

7.2

BODY MASS INDEX FOR ADULTS AGED 19 AND ABOVE (CONTINUED)

To determine your BMI, find your height in the left column. Then move across the same row to the number closest to your weight. The number at the top of that column is your BMI.

BMI	37	38	39	40	41	42	43	44	45	46	47	48	49	50	51	52	53	54
Height (inches)	Body Weight (pounds)																	
58	177	181	186	191	196	201	205	210	215	220	224	229	234	239	244	248	253	258
59	183	188	193	198	203	208	212	217	222	227	232	237	242	247	252	257	262	267
60	189	194	199	204	209	215	220	225	230	235	240	245	250	255	261	266	271	276
61	195	201	206	211	217	222	227	232	238	243	248	254	259	264	269	275	280	285
62	202	207	213	218	224	229	235	240	246	251	256	262	267	273	278	284	289	295
63	208	214	220	225	231	237	242	248	254	259	265	270	278	282	287	293	299	304
64	215	221	227	232	238	244	250	256	262	267	273	279	285	291	296	302	308	314
65	222	228	234	240	246	252	258	264	270	276	282	288	294	300	306	312	318	324
66	229	235	241	247	253	260	266	272	278	284	291	297	303	309	315	322	328	334
67	236	242	249	255	261	268	274	280	287	293	299	306	312	319	325	331	338	344
68	243	249	256	262	269	276	282	289	295	302	308	315	322	328	335	341	348	354
69	250	257	263	270	277	284	291	297	304	311	318	324	331	338	345	351	358	365
70	257	264	271	278	285	292	299	306	313	320	327	334	341	348	355	362	369	376
71	265	272	279	286	293	301	308	315	322	329	338	343	351	358	365	372	379	386
72	272	279	287	294	302	309	316	324	331	338	346	353	361	368	375	383	390	397
73	280	288	295	302	310	318	325	333	340	348	355	363	371	378	386	393	401	408
74	287	295	303	311	319	326	334	342	350	358	365	373	381	389	396	404	412	420
75	295	303	311	319	327	335	343	351	359	367	375	383	391	399	407	415	423	431
76	304	312	320	328	336	344	353	361	369	377	385	394	402	410	418	426	435	443

Source: Adapted from Clinical Guidelines on the Identification, Evaluation, and Treatment of Overweight and Obesity in Adults: the Evidence Report, 1998; The National Institutes of Health (NIH); the National Heart, Lung, and Blood Institute (NHLBI); and the National Institute of Diabetes and Digestive and Kidney Diseases (NIDDK); www.nhlbi.nih.gov/guidelines/obesity/bmi_tbl.pdf.

◄ SEE ALSO 7.4, "Underweight" ►

Although BMI can be a useful estimate of a person's body fat level, it has some weaknesses; it might overestimate body fat levels in those who have a lot of lean body mass and are muscular, and it might underestimate body fatness in those who are older and have lost muscle mass.

BMI-for-age is used to determine weight status in children. Because body fatness changes as children grow, and because girls tend to have more body fat than boys, gender and age are used to determine BMI values. Pediatricians and registered dietitians can assess children's BMIs to determine whether their body weight falls within a normal range or whether they are at risk for obesity or overweight.

Waist Circumference

Measuring your waist size is useful in both adults and children. Having more abdominal or **visceral fat** can increase your risk for diet-related diseases including cardiovascular disease, high blood pressure, and type 2 diabetes.

Waist circumference measurements are especially useful for those whose BMI is less than 35; for some populations, waist circumference helps predict the risk of chronic illness better than BMI.

Here's how to measure your waist circumference using a simple tape measure:

1. Place the tape measure snugly (but not tightly) around the bare abdomen just above the hip bone; make sure the tape measure is parallel to the floor.

2. Relax, exhale, and then measure the waist in inches.

As your waist circumference increases, so does your risk for cardiovascular and other diet-related diseases; those especially at risk include:

▶ Nonpregnant women with a waist measurement greater than 35 inches

▶ Men with a waist measurement greater than 40 inches

◀ *SEE ALSO Chapter 8, "Eat to Beat Disease"* ▶

7.2

Using a tape measure periodically to keep track of your waist size is a great way to determine how you're doing in terms of body fat level and body fat distribution.

Although there are no established norms for waist circumference in children, those who measure above the 90th percentile are more likely to have heart-disease risk factors such as higher levels of triglycerides and lower levels of HDL or good cholesterol, as well as obesity-related diseases and conditions.

◀ *SEE ALSO 7.3, "Overweight and Obesity"* ▶

Following are waist circumference values associated with higher disease risk in children.

WAIST CIRCUMFERENCE AT THE 90TH PERCENTILE IN CHILDREN (MEASURED IN CENTIMETERS)

Age in Years	Boys	Girls
2	50.8	52.2
3	54.2	55.3
4	57.6	58.3
5	61.0	61.4
6	64.4	64.4
7	67.8	67.5
8	71.2	70.5
9	74.6	73.6
10	78.0	76.6
11	81.4	79.7
12	84.8	82.7
13	88.2	85.8
14	91.6	88.8
15	95.0	91.9
16	98.4	94.9
17	101.8	98.0
18	105.2	101.0

Source: Adapted with permission from J.R. Fernandez et al., "Waist circumference percentiles in nationally representative samples of African-American, European-American, and Mexican-American children and adolescents," Journal of Pediatrics, *145 (2004): 439-444.*

A pediatrician can monitor your child's waist circumference (measured at the end of the lowest rib after your child has taken a normal breath) at her annual checkup as part of an overall health assessment.

WORDS TO GO . . . WORDS TO GO . . . WORDS TO GO

Visceral fat, also known as abdominal fat, is fat that accumulates around internal organs. This fat is more dangerous than other types of body fat because it's believed to secrete potent hormones and other chemicals that increase the risk of cardiovascular and other diseases.

7.3 OVERWEIGHT AND OBESITY

Definitions and Causes

Health Implications

How to Lose Weight

How to Maintain Weight Loss

This subchapter defines the terms overweight and obesity and discusses many causes of and the adverse health effects associated with excess body weight. It also provides tips to help you lose weight and keep it off in a safe, sensible way.

Definitions and Causes

According to the National Heart, Lung, and Blood Institute (NHLB), BMI is the common measurement used to determine weight status. Overweight, obesity, and extreme obesity are defined using BMI as follows:

▶ Overweight—BMI 25.0–29.9

▶ Obesity—BMI 30 or above

▶ Extreme obesity—BMI 40 or above

◀ *SEE ALSO 7.2, "Determining a Healthy Body Weight"* ▶

7.3

According to the most recent **National Health and Nutrition Examination Surveys** (conducted between 2005 and 2006), more than 72 million American adults—about 1 in 3 men (or 33.3 percent) and 35.3 percent of women—are currently obese. Among children between the ages of 2 and 19, 16.3 percent are obese. Although obesity rates are still quite high, there was no measurable increase in incidence between 2003 and 2004.

There are many causes of obesity and overweight. A unique interaction between genes and environment contributes to the development of overweight and obesity. For many of us, being genetically susceptible to overweight or obesity coupled with living in an environment that promotes excess consumption of high-calorie, nutrient-poor foods and beverages is destined to cause weight gain that eventually leads to overweight or obesity.

Here are some of the many factors that play key roles in the development of overweight and obesity:

▶ Increased availability of high-calorie, high-fat, and high-sugar foods and beverages that are easy to overconsume.

▶ Increased portion sizes of foods and beverages, especially those offered at restaurants, fast-food establishments, from vending machines, or wherever food is sold. People tend to consume more when offered larger portions than when offered smaller portions.

▶ More eating on the run and when distracted. People often consume more calories when they eat away from home, while driving, when listening to music, when socializing, or when otherwise on-the-go.

▶ Decreased physical activity because of unsafe neighborhoods, a lack of sidewalks or parks, and technological advances that make physical activity less of a necessity (for example, escalators, remote controls, and computers).

Health Implications

Although many people might think of overweight or obesity in terms of appearance, weighing more than what's recommended can put you at increased risk for a variety of health, psychological, and social problems. Here are some of the many adverse health consequences that are associated with a higher body weight:

▶ Coronary heart disease

▶ Type 2 diabetes

▶ Cancers (including endometrial, breast, and colon)

▶ Hypertension (high blood pressure)

▶ Dyslipidemia (high total cholesterol or high levels of triglycerides)

▶ Liver and gallbladder disease

▶ **Sleep apnea** and respiratory problems

▶ **Osteoarthritis**

▶ Gynecological problems (including menstrual problems and infertility)

Having excess body fat—especially in your abdominal area—increases the risk of type 2 diabetes, high blood cholesterol, high triglycerides, high blood pressure, and coronary artery disease.

◀ *SEE ALSO 7.2, "Determining a Healthy Body Weight"* ▷

How to Lose Weight

To lose weight, you need to create an energy deficit, or use up more calories than you consume. But before you cut calories or increase energy intake, it's important to see where you're starting from. Here are four steps you can take before you embark on weight loss:

1. Determine how many calories you need to maintain a healthy body weight.

◀ SEE ALSO 6.1, *"Estimating Your Daily Calorie Needs"* ▶

2. Find the MyPyramid daily meal pattern that's associated with your recommended calorie level (determined in step 1).

◀ SEE ALSO 6.2, *"Your Daily Meal Pattern"* ▶

3. Keep a log of everything you eat and drink (including portion sizes) for several days (including weekdays and weekend days); then compare your intake with the meal pattern that's recommended by MyPyramid (in step 2).

   A **registered dietitian (RD)** can help you assess your current intake and make recommendations for trimming your total calorie intake. She will also take into account your medical history, physical activity level, and personal preferences to help you create a lifestyle plan to help you lose weight slowly and steadily in a safe way. To find an RD in your area, contact the American Dietetic Association at www.eatright.org.

4. Keep a log of your current physical activity habits and compare it with what's recommended in current federal physical activity guidelines.

◀ SEE ALSO 7.5, *"Physical Activity and Exercise"* ▶

Before embarking on weight loss, it's important to set realistic goals. If you aim too high, you might set yourself up for disappointment. Even if you do achieve your "dream" weight, you might not be able to comfortably maintain that weight over the long term without drastically cutting back on calories and increasing physical activity and exercise. It's also important to keep in mind that it's better to lose less weight and maintain that weight loss over time than to lose a lot of weight and gain most if not all of it back. Several studies have shown that losing even 5 percent of your initial body weight (10 pounds if you weigh 200, or 7.5 pounds if you weigh 150) can significantly reduce your risk of several diet-related diseases and have health, physical, and emotional benefits.

◀ SEE ALSO Chapter 8, *"Eat to Beat Disease"* ▶

7.3

Most experts recommend a weight loss of 1–2 pounds per week. People with a higher initial body weight might shed pounds more rapidly than that, while those who start at a lower initial body weight might lose weight more slowly.

Because it takes cutting back (or burning) 3,500 calories a week to lose 1 pound of body fat, a 500-calorie deficit is needed each day. That deficit can be achieved by pairing fewer calories with more physical activity. For example, you can

> ▶ Reduce your calorie intake by 200–300 calories each day (about what's in an average candy bar or 2 slices of bread with 1 tablespoon of butter) + increase energy expenditure by 100–150 calories.

◀ *SEE ALSO 7.5, "Physical Activity and Exercise"* ▶

Simultaneously combining dietary efforts with physical activity to lose weight is smart because it supports slow, gradual weight loss and preserves lean muscle tissue to keep your metabolism revved up.

Slow and steady weight loss can also help your body adjust to a new body weight and help you stick to your new, more healthful food and fitness behaviors. On the other hand, rapid weight loss can put you at risk for developing **gallstones** and can promote rapid loss of lean muscle tissue; that slows your metabolism and makes your body less efficient at burning body fat.

Curbing Calorie Intake

Here are some tips to help you reduce your total calorie intake:

> ▶ Reduce portions of foods you typically consume, especially those that are high in calories, fat, or added sugar.

> ▶ Replace foods high in saturated and trans fats with reduced or low-fat options.

◀ *SEE ALSO 2.4, "Saturated Fats"* ▶

◀ *SEE ALSO 2.5, "Trans Fats"* ▶

◀ *SEE ALSO 8.1, "Cardiovascular Disease"* ▶

> ▶ Increase your intake of high-water, fiber-rich foods such as fruits, vegetables, whole grains, and beans; these foods take a while to eat and can help you fill up and therefore leave less room for high-calorie, low-nutrient foods.

◀ *SEE ALSO 6.4, "Vegetables"* ▶

◀ *SEE ALSO 6.5, "Grains"* ▶

◀ *SEE ALSO 6.6, "Meat and Beans"* ▶

▶ Decrease liquid calories; limit caloric beverages to low-fat or nonfat milk or soymilk, 100% fruit juice such as orange juice (up to one glass a day), and an occasional alcoholic beverage (if you are not on medications or have health conditions that preclude you from doing so).

◀ *SEE ALSO 6.3, "Fruits"* ▷

◀ *SEE ALSO 6.7, "Milk"* ▷

◀ *SEE ALSO 6.9, "Discretionary Calories"* ▷

Increasing Physical Activity and Exercise

Here are some tips to help you increase your daily energy expenditure:

▶ Find opportunities to walk more.

▶ Invest in a pedometer. Tracking the number of steps you take can be a great motivator; set a long-term goal of 10,000 steps a day and a short-term goal of increasing your daily mileage by 1,000 steps each day until you reach that goal.

▶ Instead of emailing or texting colleagues, get up and go see them or call them on the phone and walk and talk.

▶ If you don't exercise regularly at a gym or at home, identify physical activities you enjoy (whether it's dancing, ice skating, biking, or playing a sport). Set a goal to engage in that activity once a week; after you've done that for a month, add a day until you find yourself being more active several days a week.

▶ If you already go to the gym or do formal exercise, increase your frequency, intensity, or duration one or more times a week to burn more calories.

▶ Set small, reasonable goals. Sign up for a run or a charity walk alone or with a friend and use that as a great excuse to train more often and more intensely.

▶ Always check with a physician before engaging in exercise if you are pregnant or postpartum, have any medical conditions, or are on medications.

How to Maintain Weight Loss

For many people, losing weight is much easier than maintaining that weight loss long-term. But there are people who have been successful losers. The National Weight Control Registry (NWCR), a database of people who have lost significant amounts of weight and kept it off, was created by Rena Wing, Ph.D., and James O. Hill, Ph.D., from the University of Colorado. NWCR has tracked more than 5,000 of these individuals and has found the following:

▶ Registry participants have lost between 30 and 300 pounds (66 pounds on average); weight losses have been maintained for 1–66 years (5½ years on average).

▶ About half of all participants lost weight on their own, and the other half with help from some type of program.

▶ Almost all participants modified both their food intake and incorporated more physical activity to lose weight.

NWCR participants also report the following behaviors helped them keep their weight off long-term:

▶ Eating breakfast

▶ Weighing themselves at least once a week

▶ Watching less television

▶ Engaging in exercise for about an hour each day

◀ *SEE ALSO 7.5, "Physical Activity and Exercise"* ▶

▶ Eating consistently on weekdays and weekends

To lose weight and keep it off long-term, many of the behaviors that help you lose weight need to be continued to maintain weight. Many people plateau or regain weight after 6 months of cutting calories and/or increasing physical activity. But it's important to keep up the behaviors you used to lose weight in order to prevent weight regain over the long-term.

WORDS TO GO . . . WORDS TO GO . . . WORDS TO GO

National health and nutrition examination surveys are population-based surveys conducted by the National Center for Health Statistics. They are designed to assess the health and nutrition status of noninstitutionalized Americans. These surveys are currently conducted annually.

Sleep apnea is a condition in which an individual stops breathing briefly during sleep, often accompanied by snoring.

Osteoarthritis is a common form of arthritis characterized by the wearing down of cartilage (connective tissue found in many body parts) and the bone underneath it within joints.

A **registered dietitian (RD)** is a food and nutrition professional who has met American Dietetic Association (ADA) requirements; she received a Bachelor's or Master's degree in dietetics or nutrition, completed an approved internship program, passed the registration exam, and receives continuing education credits to maintain the RD credential.

Gallstones form when substances in bile (a fluid made by the liver and stored in the gallbladder) harden; they can cause pain or infection and may require surgical removal of the gallbladder.

7.4 UNDERWEIGHT

Definitions and Causes

Health Implications

How to Gain Weight

In this subchapter, you learn the definition of underweight and the potential health and other problems associated with low body weight and body fat levels. You also learn how to safely gain weight.

Definitions and Causes

Underweight is defined as having a BMI below 18.5. The World Health Organization (WHO) created the following definitions for thinness based on BMI:

▶ Mild thinness—BMI between 17 and 18.99

▶ Moderate thinness—BMI between 16 and 16.99

▶ Severe thinness—BMI below 16

◀ *SEE ALSO 7.2, "Determining a Healthy Body Weight"* ▶

Although some people can be naturally thin and still healthy, in large part because of genetic factors, some might lose weight suddenly or over time for other reasons. These include

7.4

▶ Decreased appetite due to illnesses or diseases such as **hypothyroidism,** cancer, Crohn's disease, inflammatory bowel disease, or celiac disease

▶ Decreased appetite because of medications taken for depression, high blood pressure, or osteoporosis (aspirin and some other nonsteroidal anti-inflammatory medications can also cause gastrointestinal side effects that can contribute to weight loss)

▶ Refusal to eat because of an eating disorder such as anorexia

▶ Problems chewing, tasting, or swallowing

▶ Depression, anxiety, or other psychological problems that reduce appetite

▶ Mobility problems that make it difficult to shop for and prepare meals

▶ Limited finances or lack of transportation that make food shopping and preparation difficult

Health Implications

Being underweight can contribute to symptoms such as lethargy (lack of energy), depression, and loose, elastic skin. It can also contribute to several negative health consequences, including the following:

▶ Increased risk for anemia and other nutritional deficiencies

▶ Increased risk of bone loss and osteoporosis

◀ *SEE ALSO 8.6, "Osteoporosis"* ▶

▶ Lowered immune function (which makes you more susceptible to and less able to fight off infections)

▶ Delayed wound healing

▶ Heart problems and blood vessel diseases

▶ Reduced muscle strength

▶ Reduced ability of your body to regulate temperature

▶ Increased risk of **amenorrhea** in women

If you lose weight unintentionally or experience pain or discomfort when you eat for any reason, be sure to see your physician.

How to Gain Weight

If you want or need to gain weight to make up for weight loss caused by illness, stress, or other causes, here are some tips to help you do so safely:

▶ Increase fluid intake. Drinking more low-fat milk and 100% fruit juice can provide you with valuable nutrients without filling you up.

▶ Add vegetable oils (like canola and olive oils), vegetable oil spreads, or salad dressings (made with unsaturated fats) to foods or use them to cook or prepare foods such as pasta, potatoes, lean meats and poultry, and salads.

▶ Eat nuts, seeds, and nut butters (for example, add almonds, walnuts, or sunflower seeds to salads; use pine nuts or shaved almonds to top sautéed broccoli or green beans; spread almond or peanut butter on apple slices, celery sticks, or toasted whole wheat bread).

▶ Add shredded cheese or grated Parmesan cheese to salads, potatoes, pasta, vegetable side dishes, and soups.

▶ Eat small, frequent meals. This will give you more opportunities to get key nutrients into your diet without filling you up too much.

▶ Do muscle-strengthening exercises twice a week, working all your major muscle groups.

◁ *SEE ALSO 7.5, "Physical Activity and Exercise"* ▶

WORDS TO GO . . . *WORDS TO GO . . . WORDS TO GO*

Hypothyroidism, also known as underactive thyroid, is a condition in which there is too little thyroid hormone (a hormone that keeps the metabolism revved up); symptoms might include weight gain or difficulty losing weight, constipation, hair loss, dry skin, and increased sensitivity to cold temperatures.

Amenorrhea is a condition in which a woman does not or no longer menstruates; it is caused by malfunctioning of the pituitary gland, ovaries, and uterus.

7.4

7.5 PHYSICAL ACTIVITY AND EXERCISE

Definitions and Types

Health Benefits and Risks

Weekly Recommendations

After reading this subchapter, you should understand why physical activity and exercise are important to overall health status and in helping you manage your body weight. You also learn the current weekly government recommendations for amounts and types of physical activity and exercise.

Definitions and Types

Physical activity is the umbrella term used to describe any bodily movement produced by contracting skeletal muscle that increases energy expenditure above a basal level. Exercise is physical activity that is planned, structured, and done repetitively to improve health or fitness.

The three main types of exercise are as follows:

▶ Aerobic (endurance) exercise

▶ Muscle-strengthening exercise (resistance or weight training)

▶ Bone-strengthening exercise (weight-bearing exercise)

In aerobic (or endurance) exercise, you move large muscles in your body rhythmically for a sustained period of time. This causes your heart to beat faster than usual. Examples include

▶ Brisk walking

▶ Jumping rope

▶ Running

▶ Swimming

▶ Bicycling

Three components of aerobic exercise include intensity, frequency, and duration.

When you do muscle-strengthening exercise, your muscles work or are held against a force or weight. Examples include resistance training and lifting weights.

Elastic resistance bands can be used to perform resistance exercise, as can your own body weight (to do push-ups, lunges, or squats), free weights (dumbbells or barbells), and some exercise equipment (such as a leg press machine).

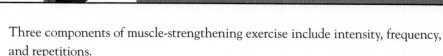
Three components of muscle-strengthening exercise include intensity, frequency, and repetitions.

Bone-strengthening exercise (also known as weight-bearing or weight-loading activity) applies force to bones to help them grow and strengthen; for example, when you walk, a force is created by impact with the ground. Examples of exercises that strengthen bones (and are also considered aerobic and muscle-strengthening) include jumping jacks, running, brisk walking, and weight-lifting.

Health Benefits and Risks

Incorporating regular exercise into your life can provide you with countless health and other benefits. Research shows that physical activity can benefit adults and children by

> ▶ Improving **cardiorespiratory fitness**

> ▶ Improving muscular fitness

> ▶ Improving bone health

> ▶ Improving cardiovascular and metabolic health biomarkers

In adults and older adults, there's strong evidence that regular physical activity

> ▶ Reduces the risk of coronary heart disease, stroke, high blood pressure, type 2 diabetes, metabolic syndrome, and some cancers (including colon and breast) as well as early death from heart disease, some cancers, and other conditions

◁ *SEE ALSO Chapter 8, "Eat to Beat Disease"* ▷

7.5

> ▶ Reduces the risk of unhealthy blood lipid levels

> ▶ Improves cardiorespiratory and muscular fitness

> ▶ Helps prevent falls that can potentially lead to fracture

> ▶ Reduces risk of depression

> ▶ Improves cognition (including thinking, learning, and judgment skills) in older people

Physical activity might also reduce symptoms of depression, improve **functional ability,** increase bone density, reduce hip fracture risk, improve the quality of sleep, and reduce the risk of lung and endometrial cancers.

Role in Weight Management

How physically active you are in general plays a key role in determining how much you weigh and how well you are able to maintain your weight over the long-term. Although engaging in aerobic or endurance-type exercise is most effective in helping you maintain your body weight, doing weights and other muscle-strengthening exercise also helps. Regular exercise can help both children and adults keep their body fat levels down (the more muscle mass you have, the more calories you burn or use up and the less body fat you have).

Being physically active, especially when you also reduce your total daily calorie intake, can create an energy deficit that leads to weight loss. Physical activity might also help reduce fat in the abdominal area (too much abdominal or visceral fat can increase the risk for heart disease and other conditions). Studies also show that for those who have lost weight, being physically active is the best way to keep weight off long-term.

◄ SEE ALSO 7.1, *"Energy Balance"* ▶

◄ SEE ALSO 7.2, *"Overweight and Obesity"* ▶

Most physical activities pose little risk for most people, but doing too much physical activity and exercise or suddenly becoming more active than usual can increase your risk for musculoskeletal injuries. Some sports, including contact sports like soccer or football, can also be associated with a higher injury risk.

Weekly Recommendations

To complement the Dietary Guidelines for Americans, in 2008 the U.S. Department of Health and Human Services (HHS) issued Physical Activity Guidelines for Americans ages 6 and above. These science-based guidelines are the first to be unveiled by the U.S. government in an effort to help Americans understand the importance of physical activity and exercise and incorporate more of it into their daily lives.

For adults and older adults without health or medical conditions that limit their mobility, both aerobic and muscle-strengthening exercise are recommended. The weekly recommendations are as follows:

▶ Aerobic exercise—2½ hours (150 minutes) at **moderate intensity** + 1¼ hours (75 minutes) at **vigorous intensity** or 1¼ hours (75 minutes) each of moderate and vigorous-intensity exercise

▶ Muscle-strengthening exercise (that works all the major muscle groups including legs, hips, back, abdomen, chest, shoulders, and arms)—2 or more days per week, but never the same muscles on back-to-back days

The weekly recommendations for aerobic and muscle-strengthening exercise are up to twice as much for adults and older adults who want to reap even more of the health benefits physical activity provides. They are

- Aerobic exercise—5 hours (300 minutes) of aerobic activity at moderate intensity; 2½ hours (150 minutes) of aerobic activity at vigorous intensity; or 2½ hours (150 minutes) each of moderate and vigorous-intensity exercise

- Muscle-strength training (that works all major muscle groups including legs, hips, back, abdomen, chest, shoulders, and arms)—2 or more days

Pregnant women are also encouraged to exercise during and after pregnancy. The weekly recommendation for pregnant women is as follows:

- Aerobic exercise—At least 2½ hours of moderate-intensity exercise spread out over an entire week

Pregnant women who already engage in vigorous activity such as running can continue with such activity but should work with their health-care provider to adjust their activity level over time. After the first trimester, pregnant women should avoid exercises in which they need to lie on their backs as well as activities that can increase the risk of falls or abdominal trauma including downhill skiing, horseback riding, soccer, and basketball. They should also avoid scuba diving because it can cause dangerous gas bubbles in the baby's circulatory system.

Here's what's recommended for children aged 6 and above:

- At least 1 hour (60 minutes) of physical activity, mostly from aerobic exercise; muscle- and bone-strengthening activities should also be included as part of the 60 minute recommendation.

Here are some examples of moderate and vigorous-intensity aerobic activities:

Moderate:

- Canoeing
- Hiking
- Skateboarding
- Rollerblading
- Biking (stationary or road bike; less than 10 miles per hour)
- Brisk walking
- Housework or yard work (sweeping, pushing a lawn mower, and so on)
- Baseball
- Softball

7.5

Vigorous:

- ▶ Fast walking
- ▶ Tag
- ▶ Flag football
- ▶ Biking
- ▶ Jumping rope
- ▶ Martial arts (such as karate)
- ▶ Running/Jogging
- ▶ Soccer
- ▶ Ice or field hockey
- ▶ Basketball
- ▶ Swimming
- ▶ Tennis
- ▶ Cross-country skiing
- ▶ Vigorous dancing
- ▶ Cross-country skiing

Source: U.S. Department of Health and Human Services (HHS), Physical Activity Guidelines, 2008.

Examples of muscle- and bone-strengthening exercises include these:

Muscle-strengthening:

- ▶ Push-ups: regular or modified (knees on floor)
- ▶ Pull-ups
- ▶ Resistance exercise using body weight or resistance bands, weight machines, or handheld weights
- ▶ Climbing (rope, tree, or wall)
- ▶ Sit-ups (curl-ups or crunches)
- ▶ Swinging on playground equipment
- ▶ Tug-of-war (and similar games)

Bone-strengthening:

- ▶ Basketball
- ▶ Gymnastics
- ▶ Hopping, skipping, and jumping (hopscotch and similar games)

▶ Jumping rope

▶ Running

▶ Tennis

▶ Volleyball

Source: U.S. Department of Health and Human Services (HHS), Physical Activity Guidelines, 2008.

The American College of Sports Medicine (ACSM) also recommends that healthy adults under the age of 65 engage in flexibility training or stretching. Stretching keeps joints limber and makes it easier to move the body. The weekly recommendation is

▶ Two to three 10- to 15-minute sessions a week; includes four repetitions for each muscle group (10–30 seconds per stretch)

The ACSM recommends doing a few minutes of aerobic exercise (such as walking for 5 minutes) before stretching to warm up muscles and minimize injury.

WORDS TO GO . . .WORDS TO GO . . .WORDS TO GO

Intensity is the amount of effort needed to perform an activity or exercise.

Frequency is how often or the number of times an activity or exercise is performed.

Duration is how long a period of time (in minutes or hours) during which an activity or exercise is performed.

Repetition refers to an exercise (for example, lifting weights or performing some other muscle-strengthening activity or exercise) that is repeated and often counted.

Cardiorespiratory fitness (also known as endurance) is a health-related component of physical fitness; it is the ability of the circulatory and respiratory systems to supply oxygen during sustained physical activity.

Functional ability is an individual's ability to perform tasks or behaviors that enable her to carry out everyday activities (for example, climbing stairs, going grocery shopping, or preparing meals at home).

Moderate-intensity physical activity is activity performed at 3–5.9 times the intensity of rest.

Vigorous-intensity physical activity is activity performed at 6 or more times the intensity of rest.

7.5

8

EAT TO BEAT DISEASE

8.1 Cardiovascular Disease

8.2 Hypertension

8.3 Diabetes

8.4 Metabolic Syndrome

8.5 Cancer

8.6 Osteoporosis

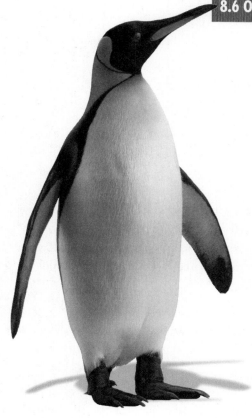

8.1 CARDIOVASCULAR DISEASE

Definitions and Causes

How to Interpret Blood Values

Diet and Lifestyle Prevention Recommendations

In this subchapter, you learn what cardiovascular diseases are and the many contributing factors. You also learn what your blood values mean and how to modify risk factors to prevent or manage various cardiovascular diseases.

Definitions and Causes

Cardiovascular disease (CVD) is an umbrella term used to describe any abnormal condition characterized by dysfunction of the heart and blood vessels (including arteries and veins).

The most common cardiovascular diseases in the United States include

▶ **Coronary heart disease** (including **myocardial infarction** or heart attack, and **angina pectoris,** or chest pain)

▶ Stroke

▶ **Heart failure**

Most cardiovascular diseases are associated with atherosclerosis, a slow and progressive process in which arteries narrow and harden. During atherosclerosis, excess amounts of fat, cholesterol, calcium, and other substances build up beneath the cells that line artery walls and contribute to the formation of **plaque.** Over time, as plaque builds up, it narrows the opening of blood vessels, limiting the amount of oxygen-rich blood and nutrients that can flow to the heart or the brain. When blood flow to the heart is blocked, a heart attack occurs; when blood flow to the brain is blocked, a stroke occurs. Harmful blood clots can also break off and block a vessel.

Although they're much less common, some forms of cardiovascular disease are caused by abnormal heart rhythm or heart valve function, or infection or toxins that make it harder for the heart to pump blood (as in **cardiomyopathy**).

Cardiovascular disease (including high blood pressure, discussed in more detail in the next subchapter) affects an estimated 81 million people in the United States. It is the leading cause of death and a major cause of disability among both men and women in the United States; it causes an estimated 700,000 deaths each year.

Although specific genes contribute to the development of some forms of cardiovascular disease (including congenital heart disease, an inherited condition present at birth), most often genetic tendencies (including family history), environment, and individual lifestyle factors interact and contribute to the development of cardiovascular diseases. Key risk factors for cardiovascular disease include

▶ High blood pressure

◀ *SEE ALSO 8.2, "Hypertension"* ▶

▶ Overweight and obesity

◀ *SEE ALSO 7.3, "Overweight and Obesity"* ▶

▶ High total or LDL cholesterol

▶ Low HDL cholesterol

▶ High triglycerides

▶ Diabetes

◀ *SEE ALSO 8.3, "Diabetes"* ▶

▶ Smoking

▶ Physical inactivity

◀ *SEE ALSO 7.5, "Physical Activity and Exercise"* ▶

How to Interpret Blood Values

A simple blood test taken after a 9- to 12-hour fast can reveal your total, LDL, and HDL cholesterol and triglyceride levels.

Because cholesterol and triglycerides cannot dissolve in blood, they are carried in the blood and throughout the body by **lipoproteins.** The three main types of lipoproteins are as follows:

▶ Low-density lipoprotein (LDL)

▶ Very low-density lipoprotein (VLDL)

▶ High-density lipoprotein (HDL)

LDL cholesterol makes up most of the cholesterol found in the blood. It is known as "bad" cholesterol because high levels indicate an unhealthy buildup

8.1

of cholesterol in the arteries; the more LDL in the blood, the greater the risk for heart disease. Too much saturated fat, trans fats, and (to a lesser extent) dietary cholesterol can contribute to high LDL levels.

◀ *SEE ALSO 2.4, "Saturated Fats"* ▶

◀ *SEE ALSO 2.5, "Trans Fats"* ▶

◀ *SEE ALSO 2.6, "Dietary Cholesterol"* ▶

HDL cholesterol, also known as "good cholesterol," carries cholesterol from other parts of the body back to the liver; the liver is in charge of moving "bad" LDL cholesterol out of the body. Having low HDL cholesterol levels increases the risk of cardiovascular disease. Consuming too little dietary fat (less than 15 percent of total calories), having high triglycerides, being overweight or obese, and having hyperglycemia or diabetes all contribute to low HDL levels.

◀ *SEE ALSO 2.1, "Functions of Fats"* ▶

◀ *SEE ALSO 7.3, "Overweight and Obesity"* ▶

Almost all the lipids found in foods and in our bodies are in the form of triglycerides (made up of a molecule of glycerol attached to three fatty acids). Having a high triglyceride level increases the risk of cardiovascular diseases. Uncontrolled diabetes, kidney or thyroid problems, or a diet that's low in protein and high in **refined carbohydrates** or alcohol can contribute to high triglyceride levels.

◀ *SEE ALSO Chapter 1, "Carbohydrates"* ▶

◀ *SEE ALSO Chapter 3, "Proteins"* ▶

◀ *SEE ALSO 6.5, "Grains"* ▶

◀ *SEE ALSO 8.3, "Diabetes"* ▶

Adults can use the table that follows to determine whether their levels of total, LDL, and HDL cholesterol and of triglycerides put them at risk for cardiovascular diseases:

TOTAL, LDL, AND HDL CHOLESTEROL AND TRIGLYCERIDE LEVELS IN ADULTS (IN MILLIGRAMS/DECILITER, MG/DL)

Total Cholesterol	
Desirable	200
Borderline High	200–239
High	≥ 240

LDL Cholesterol*	
Optimal	< 100
Near or Above Optimal	100–129
Borderline High	130–159
High	160–189
Very High	≥ 190

HDL Cholesterol**	
Protective	≥ 60
At Risk for Women	< 50
At Risk for Men	< 40

Triglycerides	
Normal	< 150
Borderline High	150–199
High	200–499
Very High	≥ 500

If you don't have coronary heart disease or diabetes and have < 1 risk factor, your LDL goal is < 160 mg/dL; with > 2 risk factors, your LDL goal is < 130 mg/dL; if you have coronary heart disease or diabetes, your LDL goal is < 100 mg/dL.

**An HDL > 60 is protective; HDL levels < 50 in women and < 40 in men are one criteria used to diagnose metabolic syndrome, a condition that increases the risk of cardiovascular and other diseases.*

Sources: Third Report of the National Cholesterol Education Program (NCEP) Expert Panel on Detection, Evaluation, and Treatment of High Blood Cholesterol in Adults (Adult Treatment Panel III) Final Report, Circulation, 2002; 106: 3143-3421; Diagnosis and Management of Metabolic Syndrome: An American Heart Association/National Heart, Lung, and Blood Institute Scientific Statement Executive Summary, Circulation, 2005; 112: 2735-2752.

8.1

A 2004 update to the National Cholesterol Education Program's (NCEP) clinical practice guidelines on cholesterol management included an even lower treatment goal of < 70 mg/dL for LDL cholesterol for very high risk people since studies have shown these lower levels to protect against heart attacks and similar coronary events. At very high risk include those with cardiovascular disease coupled with multiple or poorly controlled risk factors (such as diabetes or metabolic syndrome), or those hospitalized for heart attack or similar heart problems.

Some experts recommend using a ratio of total cholesterol to HDL cholesterol to estimate risk of cardiovascular disease. The goal is to keep your ratio below 5:1, but 3.5:1 is considered desirable. For example, someone with a total cholesterol of 175 mg/dL and an HDL of 50 would have a ratio of 3.5:1.

The AHA recommends adults aged 20 and older have their total, HDL, and LDL cholesterol and triglyceride levels measured every five years.

The **National Cholesterol Education Program (NCEP)** recommends that the following children be screened for high cholesterol starting at age 2 but no later than age 10:

▶ Those with a parent whose total cholesterol level is > 240 mg/dL

▶ Those with a family history of cardiovascular disease before age 55 in men and 65 in women

▶ Those with an unknown family history

▶ Those who are overweight or obese or have diabetes, high blood pressure, or other risk factors

You can use the following table to see how children's cholesterol and triglyceride numbers stack up:

TOTAL, LDL, AND HDL CHOLESTEROL AND TRIGLYCERIDE LEVELS IN CHILDREN (IN MILLIGRAMS/DECILITER, MG/DL)

Total Cholesterol	
Acceptable	< 170
Borderline	170–199
High	≥ 200
LDL Cholesterol	
Acceptable	< 110
Borderline	110–129
High	≥ 130
HDL Cholesterol	
Acceptable	≥ 35
Triglycerides	
Acceptable	≤ 150

Source: Report of the Expert Panel on Blood Cholesterol Levels in Children and Adolescents. National Cholesterol Education Program. National Heart Lung and Blood Institute, Public Health Service, U.S. Department of Health and Human Services, NIH Publication No. 91-2732, Bethesda, MD, September 1991.

Children with "acceptable" cholesterol levels should be rechecked in 3–5 years; those with "borderline" levels should have their levels rechecked in 1 year.

Two other measurements that can be useful in determining a person's cardiovascular risk include C-reactive protein (CRP) and homocysteine.

C-reactive protein is one of the proteins released by the body in response to an injury, an infection, or anything that causes **inflammation.** There's evidence that high CRP levels predict future heart attacks or other cardiovascular events. A blood test called a high sensitivity C-reactive protein (hsCRP) assay is currently available. This test is used with people who have already suffered from a cardiovascular "event" (e.g., heart attack, stroke) to predict their risk for additional events or in those at high risk for them. If after consulting with a doctor you decide to have your hsCRP measured, here's what your values indicate:

▶ hsCRP < 1.0 mg/L—Low risk for cardiovascular disease

▶ hsCRP between 1.0 and 3.0 mg/L—Average risk for cardiovascular disease

▶ hsCRP > 3.0 mg/L—High risk of cardiovascular disease

It's important to note that those with autoimmune diseases, cancer, or other infectious diseases can have falsely elevated hsCRP levels.

Homocysteine is an amino acid that may provide you with a glimpse of your future risk for cardiovascular disease. Recent research has linked high homocysteine levels to a greater incidence of stroke and chronic heart failure, increased death from cardiovascular disease and other adverse diseases and conditions. Although population-wide testing of homocysteine levels is not currently recommended by the American Heart Association (AHA), many researchers and practitioners believe it can be quite useful for those at high risk for cardiovascular disease; discuss it with your physician.

8.1

Diet and Lifestyle Prevention Recommendations

In 2006, the AHA created diet and lifestyle recommendations to reduce the risk for or manage cardiovascular disease in adults and children over the age of 2.

Here are some highlights of their recommendations:

▶ Balance calorie intake and physical activity to achieve or maintain a healthy body weight.

◀ SEE ALSO 7.1, *"Energy Balance"* ▶

◀ SEE ALSO 7.2, *"Determining a Healthy Body Weight"* ▶

▶ Consume a diet rich in fruits, vegetables, whole grains, and other high-fiber foods; high-fiber diets can reduce cardiovascular disease risk by decreasing cholesterol production in the body and increasing removal of harmful cholesterol from the body. High-fiber diets can also slow the progression of cardiovascular disease in those at high risk.

◀ *SEE ALSO 1.4, "Dietary Fiber"* ▶

▶ Eat fish, especially oily fish, at least twice a week (for a total of about 8 ounces); fish provides the omega-3 fats EPA and DHA, which can lower the risk of both sudden death and death from cardiovascular disease. For those with cardiovascular disease, the AHA recommends 1 gram of EPA and DHA from fish and/or fish oil supplements. For those with **hypertriglyceridemia,** the AHA recommends 2–4 grams of EPA and DHA from supplements (in capsule form). (Be sure to consult a physician before you take fish oil supplements.)

◀ *SEE ALSO 2.3, "Polyunsaturated Fats"* ▶

▶ Limit saturated fat intake to less than 7 percent of total calories, trans fat intake to less than 1 percent of total calories, and dietary cholesterol to less than 300 mg per day.

▶ Minimize intake of beverages and foods with added sugars.

▶ Choose and prepare foods with little or no sodium.

◀ *SEE ALSO Chapter 11, "Healthy Eating Tips"* ▶

▶ If you consume alcohol, do so in moderation (up to 1 drink per day for women and up to 2 drinks per day for men).

Consuming foods that are naturally rich in and enriched with **plant stanols/ sterols** can reduce the absorption of cholesterol to lower total and LDL cholesterol levels. According to the AHA, maximum effects are seen with intakes of 2 grams per day of plant stanols. Those who reduce their cholesterol levels by taking plant stanols and sterols will need to consume them each day to maintain their benefits.

◀ *SEE ALSO 10.3, "Functional Foods"* ▶

Following the previous recommendations and those of MyPyramid can reduce the risk for cardiovascular and other diet-related diseases by promoting weight loss, reducing LDL cholesterol and triglycerides, and raising HDL cholesterol.

◀ *SEE ALSO Chapter 6, "Creating a Daily Meal Plan"* ▶

◀ *SEE ALSO 8.2, "Hypertension"* ▶

◀ *SEE ALSO 8.4, "Metabolic Syndrome"* ▶

Those with diagnosed cardiovascular diseases or with risk factors such as high total and/or LDL cholesterol levels can also be prescribed medications as part of treatment, and many (or all) work more effectively when taken as part of an overall healthful dietary pattern.

WORDS TO GO . . . WORDS TO GO . . . WORDS TO GO

Coronary heart disease (CHD) is a condition in which coronary arteries, which carry blood to the heart, are narrowed so much they may slow or stop blood flow to the heart.

Myocardial infarction (MI), or heart attack, occurs when blood flow to the heart is blocked.

Angina pectoris, or angina, is chest pain that occurs when the heart can't get enough oxygen from the blood. It is a common symptom of CHD.

Heart failure resulting from a cardiac disease, which compromises ventricular systolic or diastolic function, or both. Heart failure results when the heart is unable to generate a cardiac output sufficient to meet the demands of the body without unduly increasing diastolic pressure. Heart failure can be manifested by symptoms of poor tissue perfusion alone (for example, fatigue, poor exercise tolerance, and confusion) or by both symptoms of poor tissue perfusion and congestion of vascular beds (for example, dyspnea, chest rales, pleural effusion, pulmonary edema, distended neck veins, congested liver, and peripheral edema).

Plaque is made up of cholesterol, fat, and other substances that build up on the inner walls of blood vessels.

Cardiomyopathy is a weakening or change in the structure of the heart muscle; it often manifests as inadequate heart pumping or other problems with heart function.

Lipoproteins are made up of lipids and protein; they dissolve in water and carry cholesterol through the blood and around the body either to or from blood vessels.

Refined carbohydrates are simple sugars or starches that have undergone processing.

The **National Cholesterol Education Program (NCEP)**—created in 1985 by the National Heart, Lung, and Blood Institute (NHLBI)—provides information for educators and the public to reduce the number of Americans with high blood cholesterol and prevent illness and death from CHD.

Inflammation is the body's response to injury or infection both externally and internally.

Hypertriglyceridemia is elevated blood triglycerides (blood fats).

Plant stanols/sterols are beneficial compounds found naturally in small amounts in plant foods that block cholesterol absorption.

8.1

8.2 HYPERTENSION

Definition and Causes

How to Interpret Values

Diet and Lifestyle Prevention Recommendations

In this subchapter, you learn what hypertension is and who is at risk for it. You also learn dietary and lifestyle strategies to lower your risk for or manage high blood pressure.

Definition and Causes

Blood pressure is the force of blood pushing against the walls of the arteries as the heart pumps out blood. It is measured by two numbers:

▶ Systolic blood pressure

▶ Diastolic blood pressure

When this pressure rises and stays elevated over time, it is called high blood pressure or hypertension. If not lowered, high blood pressure can damage several organs and increase the risk for heart disease, stroke, and kidney disease.

◀ SEE ALSO 8.1, *"Cardiovascular Disease"* ▶

High blood pressure affects more than 70 million Americans aged 20 and older (about 1 in 3 adults). More and more children are also developing elevated blood pressure. A recent study found almost 14 percent of boys and almost 6 percent of girls aged 8–17 had pre-hypertension; 2.6 percent of the boys and 3.4 percent of the girls already had hypertension. High blood pressure can take years to develop and, usually, those who have it experience few if any symptoms. Most cases of high blood pressure develop for unknown reasons. You can boost your odds by improving dietary and lifestyle risk factors, but some factors are out of your control. Here are both kinds of risk factors:

▶ Having a parent(s) or close relative with high blood pressure.

▶ Being African American (compared with Caucasians, African Americans often develop high blood pressure earlier and suffer more severe complications from it).

▶ Older age; the risk for high blood pressure increases for men after age 45 and for women after age 55.

▶ Being overweight or obese.

▶ Being salt-sensitive or consuming a diet high in sodium and low in potassium.

▶ Consuming a lot of alcohol.

▶ Being physically inactive.

▶ Smoking.

Chronic stress or having a disease that causes your body to retain water and/or sodium (for example, kidney disease or nervous or circulatory system problems) can also increase your risk of high blood pressure. Women who are pregnant, taking birth control pills, and on hormone replacement therapy are also at risk.

How to Interpret Values

In adults, blood pressure (measured in millimeters of mercury, mmHg) is classified into four categories based on systolic and diastolic values.

CLASSIFICATION OF BLOOD PRESSURE IN ADULTS

Classification	Systolic and Diastolic Values
Normal Blood Pressure	Systolic < 120 mmHg and Diastolic < 80 mmHg
Pre-Hypertension	Systolic of 120–139 mmHg, or Diastolic of 80–89 mmHg
Stage 1 Hypertension	Systolic of 140–159 mmHg, or Diastolic of 90–99 mmHg
Stage 2 Hypertension	Systolic of ≥ 160 mmHg, or Diastolic of ≥ 100

Source: The Seventh Report of the Joint National Committee on Prevention, Detection, Evaluation, and Treatment of High Blood Pressure (JNC 7), Hypertension. 2003;42:1206.

8.2

Any blood pressure reading at or above 120/80 mmHg increases your risk for health problems related to high blood pressure. Though 140/90 in most people is worrisome, a reading of 130/80 or higher in those with diabetes or chronic kidney disease is considered hypertension. If your systolic and diastolic numbers fall into two different categories, your classification automatically falls into the more serious category.

◀ *SEE ALSO 8.3, "Diabetes"* ▶

The NCEP recommends the following right before you have your blood pressure measured to make the results more accurate:

- ▶ Avoid coffee or cigarette smoking for 30 minutes.
- ▶ Empty your bladder before the test.
- ▶ Sit still for 5 minutes.

Children are also vulnerable to developing high blood pressure, especially as they become more overweight or obese. Your child's pediatrician can determine if your child has or is at risk for high blood pressure by taking his measurement on at least 3 separate occasions and comparing it with blood pressure standards for children based on gender, age, and height. If your child's blood pressure is at or above 120/80 mmHg, his pediatrician may determine he has pre-hypertension or hypertension (depending on how your child's values compare with norms for their gender).

Children over the age of 3 should have their blood pressure checked in a medical setting; children younger than 3 might need their blood pressure checked if they have a known kidney disease, a history of it, or other circumstance that warrant a blood pressure measurement as determined by a physician.

Diet and Lifestyle Prevention Recommendations

High blood pressure can often be prevented or treated with dietary and lifestyle changes and medications. The treatment goal is to keep blood pressure below 140/90 mmHg. For those with diabetes or kidney disease, the goal is to keep blood pressure below 130/80 mmHg.

The diet used in the Dietary Approaches to Stop Hypertension study, known as the DASH Diet, has been shown to reduce blood pressure. It emphasizes fruits, vegetables, whole grains, nuts and seeds, and low-fat dairy products. This dietary pattern is recommended by the National Institutes of Health, the AHA, MyPyramid, and the Dietary Guidelines for Americans. It is officially part of current U.S. guidelines for treating high blood pressure.

The DASH eating plan provides eating patterns for 1,600; 2,000; 2,600; and 3,100 calorie levels. Here's the plan for a standard 2,000 calorie diet:

THE DASH EATING PLAN FOR 2,000 CALORIES

Food Group	Number of Servings	Examples of One Serving
Grains*	6–8	1 slice bread; 1 ounce dry cereal**; ½ cup cooked rice, pasta, or cereal
Vegetables	4–5	1 cup raw, leafy vegetables; ½ cup cut-up raw or cooked vegetables; or ½ cup vegetable juice
Fruits	4–5	1 medium fruit; ¼ cup dried fruit; ½ cup fresh, frozen, or canned fruit
Fat-free or low-fat milk/ milk products	2–3	1 cup nonfat or low-fat milk or yogurt or 1½ ounces low-fat cheese
Lean meats, poultry, and fish	6 or less	1 ounce cooked meat, poultry, or fish; or 1 egg***
Nuts, seeds, and legumes	4–5/week	⅓ cup or 1½ ounces nuts, 2 tbsp. peanut butter, 2 tbsp. or ½ ounce seeds, ½ cup cooked dry beans or peas
Fat and oils	2–3	1 tsp. soft margarine, 1 tbsp. mayonnaise, 2 tbsp. low-fat salad dressing, 1 tbsp. regular salad dressing
Sweets	5 or less/week	1 tbsp. sugar, jelly, or jam; ½ cup sorbet or ices; 1 cup lemonade

Whole grains recommended for most grain servings.

**Equals ½–1 ¼ cups depending on cereal type.*

***Limit egg yolk intake to no more than 4 per week.*

Source: Your Guide to Lowering Blood Pressure with DASH, U.S. Department of Health and Human Services, National Institutes of Health, National Heart, Lung, and Blood Institute, NIH Publication No. 08-4082, Revised April 2006. Can be accessed at www.nhlbi.nih.gov/health/public/heart/hbp/dash/new_dash.pdf.

Other specific strategies to help you prevent high blood pressure or lower your blood pressure levels include the following:

▶ Losing weight if you're overweight or obese or preventing weight gain through reducing energy intake and increase expenditure through physical activity and exercise

◀ SEE ALSO 7.3, *"Overweight and Obesity"* ▷

◀ SEE ALSO 7.5, *"Physical Activity and Exercise"* ▷

▶ Quitting smoking and reducing exposure to secondhand smoke

▶ Learning to manage stress

▶ Reducing sodium intake

◀ *SEE ALSO 11.6, "Decreasing Sodium Intake"* ▶

▶ Increasing potassium intake

◀ *SEE ALSO 5.3, "Potassium"* ▶

WORDS TO GO . . . WORDS TO GO . . . WORDS TO GO

Systolic blood pressure is measured during a heart contraction or heart beat. It is the upper number in a blood pressure reading.

Diastolic blood pressure is measured when the heart is at rest, between contractions or beats. It is the lower number in a blood pressure reading.

8.3 DIABETES

Definition and Causes

How to Interpret Values

Diet and Lifestyle Prevention Recommendations

In this subchapter, you learn what diabetes mellitus is, the various types of diabetes, and the risk factors for each. You also learn how diabetes is diagnosed and the strategies that can reduce your risk for developing the different types of diabetes.

Definition and Causes

Diabetes mellitus, often referred to as simply diabetes, is a group of metabolic diseases characterized by hyperglycemia, or chronic high blood sugar levels. Normally, when you consume foods and beverages, your body breaks them down into glucose. That glucose then travels to your cells, and with the help of the hormone insulin, your cells absorb glucose to use for energy. When you have diabetes, however, your body is either unable to make enough insulin or to use insulin properly. Because the insulin can't usher glucose into your cells, glucose accumulates in the blood. Over time, high blood glucose levels can cause severe damage to many body organs, including the kidneys, heart, and eyes.

The American Diabetes Association (ADA) estimates that 23.6 million children and adults (or about 8 percent of the U.S. population) have diabetes, although only 18 million individuals have been diagnosed. In 2007 alone, 1.6 million new cases of diabetes were diagnosed in those aged 20 years or older.

The two main categories of diabetes include

▶ Type 1 diabetes

▶ Type 2 diabetes

Type 1 Diabetes

Type 1 diabetes, previously referred to as insulin-dependent diabetes mellitus (IDDM) or juvenile-onset diabetes, develops when the body's immune system destroys beta-cells in the pancreas. These cells are the only ones in the body that can secrete insulin. The genetic or environmental factors that cause this type of diabetes are not yet fully understood.

8.3

Type 1 diabetes can develop at any age, but it occurs most often in children and young adults. It makes up about 5–10 percent of all diagnosed cases of diabetes.

Type 2 Diabetes

Type 2 diabetes, previously called non-insulin-dependent diabetes mellitus (NIDDM) or adult-onset diabetes, usually begins as **insulin resistance,** a disorder in which the cells do not use insulin properly. As the need for insulin rises, the pancreas gradually loses its ability to produce insulin. Risk factors for type 2 diabetes include

- ▶ Older age
- ▶ Obesity
- ▶ Family history of diabetes
- ▶ History of gestational diabetes
- ▶ **Impaired glucose metabolism**
- ▶ Physical inactivity
- ▶ Race or ethnicity (African Americans, Hispanic/Latino Americans, American Indians, and some Asian Americans and Native Hawaiians or other Pacific Islanders are at particularly high risk for type 2 diabetes)

Type 2 diabetes accounts for about 90–95 percent of all diagnosed cases of diabetes. Although it occurs most often in adults, more and more children are being diagnosed with type 2 diabetes, in large part because of the increased prevalence of childhood obesity and overweight in recent decades.

Gestational Diabetes

Gestational diabetes mellitus (GDM) is **glucose intolerance** that occurs or is first recognized during pregnancy. It is estimated to occur in 1–14 percent of all pregnancies. About 5–10 percent of those who develop GDM will develop type 2 diabetes following pregnancy; those with a history of GDM have a 20–50 percent chance of developing type 2 diabetes 5–10 years after pregnancy.

Women who are most vulnerable to developing GDM are as follows:

- ▶ Those who are African American, Hispanic/Latino Americans, or American Indian
- ▶ Those who are obese
- ▶ Those with a family history of diabetes

Women with gestational diabetes need treatment to normalize their blood glucose levels to avoid complications in the fetus that can include an excessively large baby (macrosomia), injury from birth (especially if the baby is large), **hypoglycemia** after birth, or difficulty breathing.

Women who meet all of the following criteria are at low risk and do not need to be screened for GDM:

▶ Those who are under 25 years of age

▶ Those who are at a normal body weight

▶ Those with no family history (first-degree relative) of diabetes

▶ Those with no history of abnormal glucose tolerance

▶ Those with no history of poor outcomes in previous pregnancies

▶ Those who are not members of an ethnic/racial group with a high prevalence of diabetes

Other Types of Diabetes

Some types of diabetes (not classified as type 1 or type 2 diabetes) are caused by genes, excess hormones (that can result from certain diseases and conditions), drugs or chemicals, or infections. These types of diabetes account for approximately 1–5 percent of all diagnosed cases of the disease.

How to Interpret Values

According to the ADA, diabetes is diagnosed in those who meet at least one of the following criteria:

1. **Fasting Plasma Glucose** level ≥ 126 mg/dl

2. Symptoms of **hyperglycemia** and a **casual plasma glucose** level ≥ 200 mg/dl

3. 2-hour plasma glucose ≥ 200 mg/dl during an **oral glucose tolerance test**

In 2007 alone, an estimated 1 in 4 adults over the age of 20—or about 57 million Americans—had "pre-diabetes." Such individuals had either impaired fasting glucose (IFG), impaired glucose tolerance (IGT), or both. Here are the values associated with each:

▶ **impaired fasting glucose (IFG)**—A fasting plasma glucose level of 100–125 mg/dl

▶ **impaired glucose tolerance (IGT)** —A 2-hour postload glucose level of 140–199 mg/dl

8.3

223

Those with pre-diabetes are also likely to have insulin resistance, a condition during which body cells cannot use insulin properly. The pancreas produces insulin to meet the body's needs but eventually cannot make enough; this causes insulin to build up in the blood. Many people with insulin resistance have high blood levels of both glucose and insulin at the same time. Those with pre-diabetes are likely to develop type 2 diabetes within 10 years. Those with pre-diabetes and insulin resistance are also at increased risk for developing cardiovascular diseases, including coronary heart disease and stroke.

◄ SEE ALSO 8.1, *"Cardiovascular Disease"* ►

◄ SEE ALSO 8.4, *"Metabolic Syndrome"* ►

Women who are obese or have a strong family history of diabetes or personal history of GDM should be screened for the condition at their first prenatal visit. Those who are screened but do not have GDM should be retested at 24 and 28 weeks of gestation. All pregnant women at average risk for GDM (not at low risk as outlined previously) should be screened for GDM at 24–28 weeks.

To be diagnosed with gestational diabetes mellitus (GDM), a pregnant woman needs to meet one of the following criteria on two different days (unless she has already been diagnosed with hyperglycemia):

▶ Fasting plasma glucose level > 126 mg/dl

▶ Casual plasma glucose > 200 mg/dl

One of the following two approaches should be used to confirm a diagnosis of GDM in women at risk:

▶ Perform an OGTT without prior plasma or serum glucose screening.

▶ Measure plasma or serum glucose concentration 1 hour after a 50-gram oral glucose load (glucose challenge test, GCT). Those with a glucose threshold value > 140 mg/dl (7.8 mmol/l) on the GCT should then undergo an OGTT.

The values in the following table are used to diagnose GDM:

DIAGNOSIS OF GESTATIONAL DIABETES WITH A 100 G OR 75 G GLUCOSE LOAD IN AN ORAL GLUCOSE TOLERANCE TEST*:

	mg/dl	mmol/l
100 g Glucose Load		
Fasting	95	5.3
1 hour	180	10.0

	mg/dl	mmol/l
2 hour	155	8.6
3 hour	140	7.8
75 g Glucose Load		
Fasting	95	5.3
1 hour	180	10.0
2 hour	155	8.6

*Two or more of the venous plasma concentrations must be met or exceeded for a positive diagnosis; the test should be done in the morning after an overnight fast for 8–14 hours and after at least 3 days of an unrestricted diet (> 150 g carbohydrate per day) and unlimited physical activity. Subject should remain seated and should not smoke during the test.

Source: Diabetes Care, Volume 31, Supplement 1, January 2008.

Diet and Lifestyle Prevention Recommendations

Although type 1 diabetes cannot be prevented, several dietary and lifestyle strategies have been shown to reduce the risk for type 2 diabetes. For example, in the Diabetes Prevention Program, a large study of people at high risk for diabetes, participants who lost a modest 7 percent of their body weight through dietary changes (cutting calories and fat) and increased physical activity (about $2^1/_2$ hours per week) reduced their risk of developing type 2 diabetes by 58 percent.

According to the ADA, the following strategies can reduce the risk of type 2 diabetes and improve overall health:

▶ Participation in structured programs that promote moderate weight loss by reducing total calorie and dietary fat intake and engaging in regular physical activity (especially aerobic exercise)

◀ SEE ALSO 7.3, *"Overweight and Obesity"* ▷

◀ SEE ALSO 7.5, *"Physical Activity and Exercise"* ▷

▶ Consuming adequate dietary fiber and whole grains

◀ SEE ALSO 1.5, *"Daily Carbohydrate Recommendations"* ▷

◀ SEE ALSO 6.5, *"Grains"* ▷

◀ SEE ALSO 11.1, *"Increasing Fiber Intake"* ▷

▶ Consuming moderate amounts of alcohol (up to one drink per day for women and up to two drinks per day for men) for those who already drink

◀ SEE ALSO 6.9, *"Discretionary Calories"* ▷

Although there are no specific recommendations to help children reduce their risks for type 2 diabetes, the ADA suggests that healthful approaches used by adults can be applied to children as long as they meet their calorie and nutrient needs for optimal growth and development. The dietary pattern recommended by MyPyramid that emphasizes foods rich in fiber and other nutrients and minimizes saturated and trans fats, dietary cholesterol, and sodium can also be helpful.

◄ *SEE ALSO 6.1, "Estimating Your Daily Calorie Needs"* ▶

◄ *SEE ALSO 6.2, "Your Daily Meal Pattern"* ▶

The ADA and the American Dietetic Association have also created and recently expanded meal planning exchange lists. A registered dietitian (RD) or certified diabetes educator (CDE) can help you use these to plan meals and manage your diabetes. For more information, contact the ADA at 1-800-232-3472 or the American Dietetic Association at 1-800-366-1655.

WORDS TO GO . . .WORDS TO GO . . .WORDS TO GO

Insulin resistance is the body's inability to respond to and use the insulin produced by the pancreas. Insulin resistance may be linked to obesity, hypertension, and high levels of fat in the blood.

Impaired glucose metabolism refers to the state between "normal" and "diabetes" in which the risk for developing diabetes, heart attacks, and strokes is increased; two forms include impaired fasting glucose and impaired glucose tolerance.

Glucose intolerance is a pre-diabetic condition in which there is some insulin resistance causing glucose to not be able to get into cells efficiently to be used for fuel.

Hypoglycemia is an abnormally low amount of glucose or sugar in the blood.

A **fasting plasma glucose (FPG)** test measures blood sugar levels and detects problems with insulin function in the body.

Hyperglycemia is an abnormally high amount of glucose or sugar in the blood.

Casual plasma glucose is a blood glucose or blood sugar level taken at any time of the day without regard to when the last meal or snack was consumed.

An **oral glucose tolerance test** measures blood glucose level after an 8- to 16-hour fast and 2 hours after drinking a glucose-rich beverage.

8.4 METABOLIC SYNDROME

Definition and Causes

Criteria Used to Diagnose

Diet and Lifestyle Prevention Recommendations

After reading this subchapter, you should understand what metabolic syndrome is and what causes it. You learn how nutrition can play a role in the prevention or treatment and management of metabolic syndrome.

Definition and Causes

Metabolic syndrome, also known as insulin resistance syndrome, occurs when an individual has a cluster of conditions (such as hypertension) and measurements (such as a large waist size) that substantially increase his risk for cardiovascular diseases (including coronary heart disease, heart attack, and stroke) and diabetes.

◀ SEE ALSO 8.1, *"Cardiovascular Disease"* ▶

An estimated 50 million Americans have metabolic syndrome.

Several genetic, environmental, and lifestyle factors interact to create metabolic syndrome in individuals. Most at risk include those who

▶ Are overweight—have a body mass index (BMI) of > 25 and/or have abdominal obesity

◀ SEE ALSO 7.3, *"Overweight and Obesity"* ▶

▶ Engage in little physical activity

▶ Have been diagnosed with hypertension, cardiovascular disease, or **polycystic ovary syndrome (PCOS)**

◀ SEE ALSO 8.2, *"Hypertension"* ▶

▶ Have a family history of type 2 diabetes or have a personal history of gestational diabetes

◀ SEE ALSO 8.3, *"Diabetes"* ▶

▶ Are Hispanic or Asian

8.4

Criteria Used to Diagnose

Although there is no standard diagnosis for metabolic syndrome, the American Heart Association (AHA) and the National Heart, Lung, and Blood Institute adopted the criteria proposed by the National Cholesterol Education Program (NCEP) and identify metabolic syndrome in those who meet at least three of the following criteria:

- ▶ Elevated waist circumference or abdominal obesity—≥ 40 inches in men or ≥ 35 in women (≥ 32 inches in Asian women)

- ▶ High triglycerides—150 mg/dL or higher or if taking medication to treat high triglycerides

- ▶ Low HDL cholesterol—< 40 mg/dL in men and < 50 mg/dL in women or if taking medicine to raise HDL cholesterol

- ▶ Elevated blood pressure—Systolic (top number) ≥ 130 and/or diastolic (bottom number) of ≥ 85 mmHg or taking medicine to lower blood pressure

- ▶ Elevated fasting blood glucose levels—≥ 100 mg/dL

Diet and Lifestyle Prevention Recommendations

Many nutrition and lifestyle strategies used to optimize health and prevent cardiovascular disease, hypertension, and diabetes can also be used to prevent or treat metabolic syndrome and associated diseases and conditions. These include

- ▶ Weight loss if overweight, especially if you have abdominal obesity.

◀ SEE ALSO 7.2, *"Determining a Healthy Body Weight"* ▷

- ▶ Engaging in regular, consistent exercise.

- ▶ Consuming a dietary pattern consistent with MyPyramid that emphasizes fruits, vegetables, whole grains, low-fat dairy foods, fish, legumes, nuts and seeds, and healthy oils and minimizes added sugars and solid fats. It should also be rich in fiber and other key nutrients and low in saturated and trans fats, dietary cholesterol, and sodium. A Mediterranean-type diet that emphasizes plant foods and foods rich in monounsaturated fats (such as olive oil and avocados) is also a healthful option.

◀ SEE ALSO Chapter 6, *"Creating a Daily Meal Plan"* ▷

- ▶ Quitting smoking; if you are able to successfully stop smoking, make an effort to prevent weight gain by eating healthfully and engaging in regular physical activity.

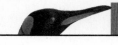

► Getting annual check-ups with a physician to determine if you have any risk factors associated with metabolic syndrome.

Following are some specific strategies to help you improve HDL cholesterol and triglyceride levels as well as blood pressure (and therefore reduce your risk for metabolic syndrome and other diet-related diseases and conditions).

Raising HDL Cholesterol Levels

You can raise HDL or "good" cholesterol levels by:

► Losing weight

◄ *SEE ALSO 7.3, "Overweight and Obesity"* ►

► Increasing aerobic exercise

◄ *SEE ALSO 7.5, "Physical Activity and Exercise"* ►

► Emphasizing foods rich in monounsaturated and polyunsaturated fats over those rich in saturated and trans fats

◄ *SEE ALSO 2.3, "Polyunsaturated Fats"* ►

◄ *SEE ALSO 11.3, "Decreasing Saturated Fat Intake"* ►

◄ *SEE ALSO 11.4, "Decreasing Trans Fat Intake"* ►

► Quitting smoking

► Drinking moderately (having up to one drink a day for women and up to two drinks a day for men) if you already drink

Lowering Triglycerides

8.4

You can lower your blood triglyceride level by:

► Taking 2–4 grams of fish oil supplements (in capsule form); be sure to discuss this with your physician first

► Emphasizing foods rich in monounsaturated and polyunsaturated fats over those rich in saturated and trans fats

◄ *SEE ALSO 2.2, "Monounsaturated Fats"* ►

◄ *SEE ALSO 2.3, "Polyunsaturated Fats"* ►

► Replacing refined grains with whole grains and reducing your intake of foods and beverages rich in simple sugars and low in nutrients (such as soda and candy)

◁ SEE ALSO 11.1, *"Increasing Fiber Intake"* ▷

◁ SEE ALSO 11.2, *"Decreasing Added Sugar Intake"* ▷

▶ Avoiding alcohol

▶ Avoiding cigarette smoking

Lowering Blood Pressure

You can lower your blood pressure by:

▶ Losing weight

◁ SEE ALSO 7.3, *"Overweight and Obesity"* ▷

▶ Reducing sodium intake

◁ SEE ALSO 8.2, *"Hypertension"* ▷

◁ SEE ALSO 11.6, *"Decreasing Sodium Intake"* ▷

▶ Increasing potassium intake

◁ SEE ALSO 5.3, *"Potassium"* ▷

WORDS TO GO . . . WORDS TO GO . . . WORDS TO GO

Polycystic ovary syndrome (PCOS) is a condition (possibly inherited) that involves menstrual irregularities and elevated levels of androgens (male hormones) in women with no other diseases. Symptoms can include multiple ovarian cysts, amenorrhea, failure of ovaries to release eggs (anovulation), excess body hair, a high rate of miscarriage, and/or infertility.

8.5 CANCER

Definitions and Causes

Diet and Lifestyle Prevention Recommendations

In this chapter, you learn what cancer is and the key factors that contribute to its development. You also learn how diet and lifestyle can reduce your risk for developing cancer.

Definitions and Causes

Cancer is the general term used to describe diseases in which cells that control growth and normal body functions become damaged and divide without control and invade other body tissues. Normally, the body creates new cells to replace old ones that die. Sometimes, new cells grow when you don't need them and old cells don't die. These extra cells can create a mass called a *tumor*. Tumors can be benign (noncancerous) or malignant (cancerous). Sometimes cancer spreads from one part of the body to another in a condition called *metastasis*.

According to the National Cancer Institute (NCI), approximately 10.7 million Americans were living with cancer in 2005 (the most recent year that provided good estimates of this information). The American Cancer Society (ACS) estimated that in 2008, more than 1.4 million new cancer cases were expected to be diagnosed. Although there are more than 100 types of cancer, the most prevalent in the United States include, from most to least, the following:

▶ Breast cancer

▶ Prostate cancer

▶ Colon and rectal cancer

▶ Melanoma of skin

▶ Urinary bladder

▶ Endometrial cancer and uterine sarcoma

Although all cancers involve malfunctions of **genes** involved in cell growth and division, only 5 percent of all cases are inherited; most cancers result from damage or mutation of genes caused by individual factors or the interaction of several factors. According to the NCI, the most common nongenetic risk factors for cancer include

8.5

▶ Aging

▶ Tobacco use

▶ Exposure to ultraviolet rays from the sun and other sources

▶ Ionizing radiation (from x-rays and other sources)

▶ Certain chemicals, biological agents, and other substances

▶ Some viruses and bacteria

▶ Certain hormones

▶ Drinking more than two alcoholic beverages every day for many years

▶ Poor diet, lack of physical activity, or being overweight

Diet and Lifestyle Prevention Recommendations

Like many diseases, cancer is caused by a combination of genetic, environmental, and lifestyle factors, making its prevention a challenge. Nevertheless, the ACS estimates that making healthful dietary and lifestyle changes can prevent up to one third of all cancers. Several governmental and other organizations (including the ACS, the NCI, and others) have developed dietary and lifestyle recommendations and guidelines to help Americans substantially reduce their risks for developing cancer. These recommendations include the following:

▶ Achieving and maintaining a healthier or healthy weight (and avoiding unhealthy weight gain throughout life) by balancing calorie intake with physical activity.

◀ SEE ALSO 7.2, *"Determining a Healthy Body Weight"* ▶

▶ Adopting a physically active lifestyle that includes regular exercise.

◀ SEE ALSO 7.5, *"Physical Activity and Exercise"* ▶

▶ Eating a variety of healthful foods, especially plant foods.

◀ SEE ALSO 6.2, *"Your Daily Meal Pattern"* ▶

▶ Choosing whole grains over refined grains and foods made with added sugars.

◀ SEE ALSO 6.5, *"Grains"* ▶

◀ SEE ALSO 6.9, *"Discretionary Calories"* ▶

◀ SEE ALSO 11.1, *"Increasing Fiber Intake"* ▶

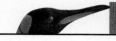

▶ Limiting consumption of processed and red meats; they contain **nitrates** and other **carcinogens.**

◀ *SEE ALSO 11.3, "Decreasing Saturated Fat Intake"* ▶

▶ If you drink alcoholic beverages, limiting intake. Alcohol is an established cause of cancers of the mouth, pharynx, larynx, esophagus, and liver and can also play a role in breast and colorectal cancer.

Those who are at average risk for cancer and who have no specific symptoms can get screening guidelines for a variety of cancers at www.cancer.org/docroot/ped/content/ped_2_3x_acs_cancer_detection_guidelines_36.asp.

WORDS TO GO . . . WORDS TO GO . . . WORDS TO GO

Genes are basic units of heredity (transmission of genes from parent to child) made of deoxyribonucleic acid (DNA).

Nitrates are preservatives that add flavor and color to cured meats such as hot dogs and bacon.

Carcinogens are substances that cause cancer.

8.5

8.6 OSTEOPOROSIS

Definitions and Causes

Diet and Lifestyle Prevention Recommendations

In this subchapter, you learn what osteoporosis is and the various factors that contribute to its development. You also learn dietary and lifestyle strategies that can help you lower your risk for osteoporosis.

Definitions and Causes

Osteoporosis is a skeletal disease in which bones gradually lose mass, become less dense, and weaken over time. This increases the risk for bone fractures, which can impair mobility or lead to severe consequences such as death. Often osteoporosis develops over many years; because there are usually no symptoms associated with the condition, osteoporosis often goes undetected until a fracture occurs.

According to the National Osteoporosis Foundation (NOF), an estimated 10 million Americans currently have osteoporosis and another 34 million have osteopenia (low bone mass). By 2010, the NOF estimates those numbers will increase to 12 million and 40 million, respectively. The NOF also estimates that 1 in 2 women and 1 in 4 men above the age 50 will experience a fracture related to osteoporosis sometime in their lives.

Normally, bones go through periods in which they grow and are broken down at a constant rate throughout life. During childhood and adolescence, bone mass increases more rapidly than it's lost, and by age 30, people achieve **peak bone mass.** After this, bone loss occurs slowly over time, but outpaces the rate at which it is formed.

Although genetics play a key role in peak bone mass, (the total amount of bone formed in a person's body), several other factors contribute to one's risk of developing osteoporosis. Most at risk are

- ▶ Those who have a thin, small frame
- ▶ Those with a family history of osteoporosis
- ▶ Women who are postmenopausal, who went through early menopause, or who have amenorrhea
- ▶ Women who are white or Asian

▶ Men with low levels of **testosterone**

▶ Those who have osteopenia

Some people who develop osteoporosis have no obvious risk factors, and some develop the condition as a consequence of taking medications for a variety of diseases and conditions.

Some other factors that also increase the risk for osteoporosis include

▶ Not consuming enough calcium from foods or supplements

▶ Inactivity (due to bed rest or limited mobility) or otherwise engaging in low levels of physical activity

▶ Consuming too much alcohol

Diet and Lifestyle Prevention Recommendations

Although there's no cure, osteoporosis is a disease that is highly preventable in most situations. Here are some steps you can take to reduce your risk for osteoporosis:

▶ Maintain a healthy body weight.

◀ *SEE ALSO Chapter 7, "Weight Management"* ▷

▶ Get adequate calcium and vitamin D from the diet or supplements. Calcium is an essential mineral for building strong bones and attaining a high peak bone mass, and vitamin D helps the body absorb calcium. Together, calcium and vitamin D can help retard bone loss and reduce fracture risk even in those who already have osteoporosis.

◀ *SEE ALSO 4.3, "Vitamin D"* ▷

◀ *SEE ALSO 5.5, "Calcium"* ▷

▶ Engage in regular physical activity, including weight-bearing and bone- and muscle-strengthening exercises; weight-bearing exercises help your body work against gravity to strengthen bones, and muscle-strengthening exercises can promote agility and strength and reduce your risk for falls.

▶ Limit or eliminate alcohol from the diet. Even small amounts of alcohol (2–3 ounces) can damage bones, and too many calories from alcohol can displace calories from nutrient-dense foods and beverages and reduce overall nutrition status.

◀ *SEE ALSO 6.9, "Discretionary Calories"* ▷

8.6

▶ If you smoke, stop; smoking reduces calcium absorption and can lead to early menopause (during menopause, the hormone estrogen, which helps preserve bones, is reduced substantially).

▶ Have your bone mineral density tested. A dual energy x-ray absorptiometry (DXA) test measures bone density at various sites in the body and predicts future bone fracture risk.

Some at risk for or who develop osteoporosis can need medications to prevent or treat the condition and should discuss the various options with a physician.

WORDS TO GO . . . *WORDS TO GO* . . . *WORDS TO GO*

Peak bone mass is the maximum bone density and strength developed in individuals by age 30.

Testosterone is a sex hormone (or androgen) produced by the testes that contributes to the development of male sex characteristics, including a deep voice and facial hair. It also strengthens muscles and bones.

9

FOOD ALLERGIES, INTOLERANCES, AND SENSITIVITIES

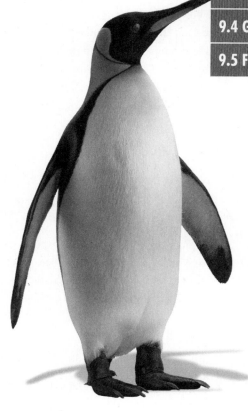

9.1 FOOD ALLERGIES

Definition, Causes, and Symptoms

Common Food Allergens

Prevention and Treatment

This chapter provides an overview of food allergies, including their causes and symptoms. Common food allergens and tips on how to avoid or treat allergic reactions are also discussed.

Definition, Causes, and Symptoms

A true food allergy is a heightened response of the immune system to a food or food component. When someone with a true food allergy ingests a food or food component to which they are allergic, the body's immune system labels it as a foreign invader. To defend against the perceived threat, the immune system commands the body to produce large amounts of proteins called immunoglobulin (IgE) antibodies. The antibodies attach themselves to specific cells called mast cells, which triggers the release of **histamine** and other chemicals into the bloodstream. It's these chemicals that cause a variety of symptoms in several parts of the body.

◀ *SEE ALSO 12.2, "Other Harmful Substances in Food"* ▶

According to the **Food Allergy and Anaphylaxis Network (FAAN)**, approximately 12 million people in the United States (about 4 percent of the population) have food allergies. The FDA estimates food allergies cause 30,000 emergency room visits and 150 deaths each year.

People at risk for food allergies include those whose parents had any kind of allergies, including hay fever and asthma, and those whose mothers smoked during pregnancy. But people without a family history of allergies can develop them, too.

Food allergies often become apparent during early childhood, but they can also emerge in later childhood and even in adulthood.

Allergy symptoms appear anywhere from a few minutes to two hours after being exposed to a food allergen. Response times differ from person to person and can vary even in individuals exposed to the same allergen on different occasions. Symptoms can be mild or severe and can include the following.

▶ Flushed skin or skin irritations such as hives, rashes, or eczema

▶ Tingling or itchiness in the mouth

▶ Swelling in the face, tongue, lips, throat, or vocal chords

▶ Gastrointestinal symptoms such as stomach cramps, diarrhea, or vomiting

▶ Wheezing or breathing problems

▶ Coughing, sneezing, or a runny nose

▶ Dizziness or lightheadedness

People who have both food allergies and asthma are especially vulnerable to developing a severe reaction when exposed to a food allergen. **Anaphylaxis,** a life-threatening condition, can occur very quickly after exposure to a food allergen. It can affect several body parts at the same time, causing blocked airways in the lungs, extremely low blood pressure and anaphylactic shock, or a swelled throat that can lead to suffocation. Of all food allergens, peanuts and tree nuts typically cause the most severe symptoms.

If you or one of your children experiences symptoms after eating a particular food, be sure to speak with a physician or a board-certified allergist (if possible, while experiencing symptoms), as subsequent exposures might produce a more severe reaction.

Your doctor can recommend any combination of an **elimination diet,** skin tests, blood tests, or a double-blind placebo-controlled food challenge (to verify the diagnosis).

Common Food Allergens

Although more than 160 foods can trigger food allergies, the following are the most common food allergens in the United States:

▶ Milk

▶ Tree nuts (including almonds, walnuts, pecans, cashews, Brazil nuts, pistachios, hazelnuts, pine nuts, macadamia nuts, chestnuts, and hickory nuts)

▶ Peanuts

▶ Soybeans

▶ Wheat

▶ Egg

9.1

- ▶ Crustacean (including shrimp, crab, lobster, and crayfish)
- ▶ Fish (including all species of finfish such as bass, flounder, and cod)

Less common but still notable:

- ▶ Certain fruits
- ▶ Vegetables (such as celery)
- ▶ Seeds (such as sesame, poppy, or sunflower)
- ▶ Buckwheat
- ▶ Legumes
- ▶ Mollusks (such as clams and oysters)

Some people can have a cross-reactivity food allergy in which one food or plant allergy causes them to be allergic to other similar foods. For example, people allergic to cashews or to natural rubber latex may develop a cross-reactivity allergy to mangoes, because of similar antigens in the plants. Most individuals who have a food allergy are also allergic to dust or have other allergies unrelated to food.

Prevention and Treatment

Although exclusive breastfeeding can delay or prevent the onset of food allergies in infants, there is currently no known cure for or established way to prevent food allergies from developing altogether. Although allergies to peanuts, tree nuts, and fish often persist throughout life, many children allergic to milk, soybeans, wheat, or eggs eventually outgrow these allergies.

According to American College of Allergy, Asthma, and Immunology (ACAAI) recommendations, parents of infants who have a family history of allergies of any kind should wait until their infants are at least 6 months old before introducing solid foods. The following food introduction timeline is also recommended:

- ▶ Dairy products—12 months of age
- ▶ Hen's eggs—24 months of age
- ▶ Peanuts (including peanut butter), tree nuts, fish, and seafood—36 months of age (or later)

Because soybeans and wheat are also common allergens, the ACAAI recommends speaking with a pediatrician to determine when those foods can be introduced. A registered dietitian can help parents create appropriate meal plans for their children to ensure they're getting all the key nutrients needed to support optimal growth and development.

The ACAAI also advises that infants and children who don't appear to be at risk for allergies not be given solid foods until at least 6 months of age and to offer potential food allergens (including eggs, peanuts/peanut butter, tree nuts, fish, and seafood) one at a time and with caution to help parents better identify an allergic reaction if it does occur.

For those who have food allergies, avoiding allergenic foods (and foods processed or prepared with them) is critical because even tiny amounts of an offending food can trigger a severe or fatal reaction. Fortunately, since 2006, the Food Allergen Labeling and Consumer Protection Act (FALCPA) has required food manufacturers to state simply and clearly on food and beverage packages the food source of the eight "major food allergens" (milk, tree nuts, peanuts, soybeans, wheat, egg, crustacean shellfish, and fish). These are responsible for 90 percent of all food allergies that occur in the United States.

Ingredients (including flavorings, colorings, or any other food additives) that contain proteins derived from any of these foods must also be clearly labeled on food and beverage packages.

If the food source of a "major food allergen" is not part of an ingredient's common or usual name or is not already listed on the ingredients list, it can appear in the ingredients list in parentheses after the name of the ingredient. For example:

- ▶ whey (milk)
- ▶ lecithin (soy)
- ▶ flour (wheat)
- ▶ enriched flour (wheat flour) and so on

Another option is to put a "Contains" statement immediately after or next to the ingredients list. For example

Contains Wheat, Milk, Eggs, and Soy

Because the statements "can contain" and "free" are not defined by the FDA for use on food packages, it's better to err on the side of caution and avoid such foods unless you've been assured by the manufacturer that the product does not contain any ingredients to which you're allergic.

9.1

It's very important that individuals with food allergies, including those allergic to foods that don't need to be declared on food packages (such as sesame seeds), carefully read a product's ingredient list before consuming the food. Because food labels are not available when eating away from home, at outings, at events, or in restaurants and labels (and allergen labeling) are not required for fresh produce, meat, and some highly refined oils, it's critical to be careful when choosing any foods that are not labeled and make sure they're prepared in a way that protects them from contamination with allergens.

It's also important to keep checking the labels of foods and beverages you regularly consume because manufacturers often change their packaging or ingredients; if you're unsure whether a particular packaged food is safe to eat, contact the manufacturer.

◀ *SEE ALSO 10.1, "Reading Food Labels"* ▶

Those with food allergies should always have an epinephrine autoinjector (such as an EpiPen or Twinject) on hand with instructions for others should they experience a severe reaction and require help with a lifesaving injection. Wearing a medical alert bracelet or carrying a card in your wallet or purse that indicates you have a food allergy can also be helpful.

WORDS TO GO . . .WORDS TO GO . . .WORDS TO GO

Histamine is a powerful chemical found in some of the body's cells and produced by the breakdown of histidine, an amino acid. It is responsible for many of the symptoms experienced by those with allergies to foods, dust, or other substances and can cause a variety of symptoms that affect the eyes, nose, throat, lungs, skin, or gastrointestinal tract. Histamine can be found in improperly stored fish, and in some cheeses, fermented soy products, sauerkraut, alcoholic beverages, and vinegars.

Food Allergy and Anaphylaxis Network (FAAN) is a nonprofit organization of more than 30,000 consumers, health professionals, government representatives, and others worldwide. It raises awareness of, provides resources for, and enhances the understanding of food allergies and anaphylaxis.

Anaphylaxis is a severe systemic reaction (involving many body systems) caused by the immune system after consumption of an allergenic food or food component. It can cause you to stop breathing.

An **elimination diet** is a diet that is used to identify a food or food component that prompts an allergic response in an individual. Foods that appear to cause problems are removed from the diet one by one until the one that causes the symptoms is identified.

9.2 FOOD ADDITIVE SENSITIVITIES

Overview

Monosodium Glutamate

Sulfites

FD&C Yellow #5

Aspartame

Caffeine

In this subchapter, you learn what food additives are and some common additives that can elicit adverse reactions in some individuals.

Overview

Food additives are ingredients added to foods to preserve flavor, enhance texture, provide color, maintain or improve their safety, or improve or preserve their nutritional value. Food additives include any and all substances used to produce, process, treat, package, transport, or store foods.

Thousands of ingredients are legally added to foods, and the FDA has created a database called "Everything Added to Food in the United States" that lists 3,000 ingredients that have been approved as food additives by the FDA or that are listed as **generally recognized as safe (GRAS).**

All food additives must be considered safe at their intended level of use before they can be added to foods, and are subjected to ongoing safety reviews. They must also meet Good Manufacturing Practices (GMP) that limit amounts of a food or color additive that can be used to the amount needed to achieve the desired effect.

Monosodium Glutamate

9.2

Monosodium glutamate (MSG) is a salt of the amino acid glutamic acid. It's used as a flavor enhancer and is found in a variety of foods including processed foods such as canned vegetables, canned tuna, salad dressings, and many frozen foods and in many restaurant foods including Chinese food. Glutamate is also found naturally in some foods (including tomatoes and Parmesan cheese), although no adverse symptoms have been reported from consumption of these foods according to the Centers for Science in the Public Interest (CSPI).

◀ *SEE ALSO 3.1, "Functions of Protein"* ▷

The FDA and the Federation of American Societies for Experimental Biology have reviewed the scientific data on possible adverse reactions that can occur in response to glutamate. Although most people can safely consume MSG, a GRAS substance, a small number of people can experience negative side effects quickly after consuming MSG-containing foods. Symptoms can include ...

▶ Flushing

▶ Warm sensations in the back of the neck or forearms

▶ Headache

▶ Nausea

▶ Chest discomfort

▶ Feelings of detachment

Those who think they are sensitive to MSG and those who follow low-sodium diets for hypertension or other diseases or conditions should avoid MSG. It will be listed on the ingredient list as "monosodium glutamate"; glutamate can also be found in **"hydrolyzed protein"** or "natural flavorings." If in doubt, you can call the food manufacturer to see whether the product contains MSG.

◀ *SEE ALSO 5.2, "Sodium"* ▶

◀ *SEE ALSO 8.2, "Hypertension"* ▶

◀ *SEE ALSO 10.1, "Reading Food Labels"* ▶

Sulfites

Sulfites are **preservatives** used primarily as an antioxidant in a variety of foods to prevent browning and to maintain the color of foods such as dried fruit, "fresh" shrimp, golden raisins, and processed potatoes. They're used to inhibit the growth of bacteria in fermented foods such as wine and can be added to medications to increase shelf life.

Other foods that can contain sulfites include the following.

FDA GUIDE TO FOODS AND DRUGS WITH SULFITES*

Food Category	Type of Food
Alcoholic beverages	Beer, cocktail mixes, wine, wine coolers
Baked goods	Cookies, crackers, mixes with dried fruits or vegetables, pie crust, pizza crust, quiche crust, flour tortillas
Beverage bases	Dried citrus fruit beverage mixes
Condiments and relishes	Horseradish, onion and pickle relishes, pickles, olives, salad dressing mixes, wine vinegar
Confections and frostings	Brown, raw, powdered, or white sugar derived from sugar beets
Modified dairy products	Filled milk (a specially prepared skim milk in which vegetable oils, rather than animal fats, are added to increase its fat content)
Drugs	Anti-emetics (taken to prevent nausea), cardiovascular drugs, antibiotics, tranquilizers, intravenous muscle relaxants, analgesics (painkillers), anesthetics, steroids and nebulized bronchodilator solutions (used for treatment of asthma)
Fish and shellfish	Canned clams; fresh, frozen, canned, or dried shrimp; frozen lobster; scallops; dried cod
Fresh fruit and vegetables	Sulfite use banned (except for fresh potatoes)
Gelatins, puddings, and fillings	Fruit fillings, flavored and unflavored gelatin, pectin jelling agents
Grain products and pastas	Cornstarch, modified food starch, spinach pasta, gravies, hominy, breadings, batters, noodle/rice mixes
Jams and jellies	Jams and jellies
Nuts and nut products	Shredded coconut
Plant protein products	Canned, bottled, or frozen fruit juices (including lemon, lime, grape, and apple); dried fruit; canned, bottled, or frozen dietetic fruit or fruit juices; maraschino cherries and glazed fruit

9.2

continues

FDA GUIDE TO FOODS AND DRUGS WITH SULFITES* (CONTINUED)

Food Category	Type of Food
Processed vegetables	Vegetable juice, canned vegetables (including potatoes), pickled vegetables (including sauerkraut), dried vegetables, instant mashed potatoes, frozen potatoes, potato salad
Snack foods	Dried fruit snacks, trail mixes, filled crackers
Soups and soup mixes	Canned seafood soups, dried soup mixes
Sweet sauces, toppings and syrups	Corn syrup, maple syrup, fruit toppings, high-fructose corn syrup, pancake syrup
Tea	Instant tea, liquid tea concentrates

*The above foods and drugs CAN contain sulfites, according to the FDA. Not all manufacturers use sulfites in these products, and the amounts can vary. Remember to check the product label.

Source: FDA, edis.ifas.ufl.edu/FY731.

Although most people can safely consume sulfites, the FDA acknowledges that about 1 of every 100 people in the United States, especially those with asthma, is sensitive to these additives. Sulfite-containing foods give off a gas called sulfur dioxide. When a person with asthma eats such foods, she inhales the gas, which irritates and constricts her lungs,, making breathing very difficult.

Sulfite ingestion can cause the following symptoms in those who are sensitive:

- ▶ Anaphylactic shock

- ▶ Hives

- ▶ Angioedema (swelling beneath the skin)

- ▶ Nausea

- ▶ Abdominal pain

- ▶ Diarrhea

- ▶ Seizures

Since 1986, the FDA has prohibited sulfite use on fresh produce sold or served raw to consumers. Although still used in a variety of processed foods, sulfites must be listed on food labels. If you see any of the following terms in an ingredient list, it means the product contains sulfites:

- ▶ Sulfur dioxide

- ▶ Sodium sulfite

- ▶ Sodium or potassium bisulfite

- ▶ Sodium or potassium metabisulfite

FD&C Yellow #5

FD&C Yellow 5, also known as tartrazine, is a widely used synthetic additive that colors beverages, gelatin dessert, candy, baked goods, ice creams, custards, and some medications. Although the FDA regulates color additives to ensure they are safe to consume, a very small proportion of the U.S. population (about 0.1–0.1 percent) is sensitive to this food dye, especially those with asthma, those sensitive to aspirin, and those who take aspirin regularly.

Individuals with this sensitivity can experience symptoms such as the following:

▶ Hives

▶ Purpura (purple skin bruising)

▶ Anaphylaxis or anaphylactic shock

Since 1981, the FDA has required all foods containing FD&C Yellow 5 to list the additive on all ingredient labels.

Aspartame

Aspartame is an artificial, low-calorie sweetener made of aspartic acid and phenylalanine, two amino acids, and methanol. It is found in a variety of foods and beverages including diet sodas and other beverages, yogurt, pudding, gelatin desserts, and chewing gum. It's also sold as the tabletop sweeteners NutraSweet and Equal.

Aspartame is 200 times sweeter than sucrose (a simple sugar) and is used in such small amounts in foods that it's virtually calorie free. It was first approved by the FDA for use in low-calorie tabletop sweeteners and powdered mixes in 1981, and in all foods and beverages since 1996.

◀ *SEE ALSO 10.4, "Fat Replacers and Sugar Substitutes"* ▶

Despite aspartame's approval by the FDA, some people have reported a wide range of symptoms associated with consumption of aspartame-containing foods and beverages, such as headaches, dizziness, mood changes, vomiting, nausea, and many others. Despite this, the FDA deems aspartame safe for use by the general public, including those with diabetes, pregnant and nursing women, and children. This conclusion is consistent with that of several other organizations that have also reviewed extensive research on aspartame, including the American Medical Association, the American Diabetes Association, and the American Dietetic Association.

9.2

The **acceptable daily intake (ADI)** for aspartame, set by the FDA, is 50 milligrams per kilogram (mg/kg) of body weight. To reach the ADI, an adult would need to consume any of the following on a typical day (in approximate amounts):

▶ 20 cans of diet soda

▶ 42 servings of sugar-free gelatin

▶ 97 packets of low-calorie tabletop sweeteners

Despite its safety for most people, some people are unable to properly metabolize phenylalanine, an essential amino acid. This can lead to an unhealthy buildup of the amino acid in the body. People who need to severely restrict their intake of aspartame (which contains phenylalanine) include

▶ Those with **phenylketonuria (PKU),** a rare inherited disease

▶ Pregnant women with hyperphenylalanine (high levels of phenylalanine in their blood)

Products made with aspartame are required by law to have a warning label that says they contain phenylalanine to alert those with PKU who need to avoid the substance.

Caffeine

Caffeine is a bitter substance found naturally in the leaves, seeds, and fruits of plants. It is naturally found in coffee, tea, cocoa and cocoa products, and some flavorings. It's also added to a variety of foods including carbonated beverages, energy drinks, chocolate-flavored milks, yogurts, frozen desserts, and even some medicines such as over-the-counter pain-relievers.

Up to 300 milligrams a day (the amount of caffeine in about three cups of brewed coffee) is considered safe for most people. Although caffeine is classified as GRAS by the FDA, some people can be sensitive to its effects. Symptoms include

▶ Insomnia

▶ Headaches

▶ Irritability

▶ Nervousness

▶ Migraine headaches

The effects of caffeine intake on individuals can vary and depend on many factors, such as body weight, how much is consumed, how often it's consumed, and overall health status. Children, for example, tend to be a lot more sensitive to the effects of caffeine than adults. Those who experience symptoms should limit or avoid caffeine, as should the following:

▶ Those with heartburn

▶ Those who have peptic ulcers

▶ Those who suffer from anxiety or panic attacks

▶ Those with a history of depression or who take antidepressant medications

Because caffeine content is not required to be listed on food and beverage packages, calling the manufacturer is the best way to determine how much caffeine a product contains. Here are some estimates for the amount of caffeine in some common foods and beverages:

ESTIMATED AMOUNTS OF CAFFEINE IN FOODS AND BEVERAGES

Food or Beverage	Milligrams (mg)	Typical Range
8 oz. (1 cup) coffee:		
Brewed, drip method	85	65–120
Instant	75	60–85
Decaffeinated	3	2–4
Espresso (1 oz. cup)	40	30–50
8 oz. (1 cup) tea:		
Brewed, major U.S. brands	40	20–90
Brewed, imported brands	60	25–110
Instant	28	24–31
Iced	25	9–50
Some soft drinks (12 oz.)	36	0–71*
Cocoa beverage (8 oz.)	6	3–32
Chocolate milk (8 oz.)	5	2–7
Milk chocolate (1 oz.)	6	1–15
Dark chocolate, semisweet (1 oz.)	20	5–35
Baker's chocolate	26	26
Chocolate-flavored syrup	4	4

Sources: "Everything You Need to Know About Caffeine," International Food Information Council.

*Centers for Science in the Public Interest, "Caffeine Content of Food and Drugs," September 2007; www.cspinet.org/new/cafchart.htm.

9.2

Generally recognized as safe (GRAS) is a term created by the FDA that indicates a chemical or substance added to food is considered safe under conditions of its intended use.

Hydrolyzed proteins are proteins that have been chemically broken down in the body into amino acids. When these proteins are broken down, glutamate is formed and joins with free sodium to form MSG.

A **preservative** helps maintain the freshness of food; protects against spoilage by organisms such as bacteria, molds, fungi, and yeasts; and slows or prevents changes in color, flavor, and textures of food.

Acceptable daily intake (ADI) is an estimate of how much of a substance can be consumed over a lifetime without significant health risk. It is often used for food additives.

Phenylketonuria (PKU) is an inherited condition in which the body cannot process phenylalanine, an essential amino acid, because it lacks or does not have enough of the enzyme called PKU which, if left untreated, can cause irreversible mental retardation, small head size, epilepsy, or behavioral problems.

9.3 LACTOSE INTOLERANCE

Definition and Causes

Symptoms

Dietary Treatment

In this subchapter, you learn the causes, symptoms, and dietary treatment strategies for lactose intolerance, a common food intolerance in the United States.

Definition and Causes

Lactose intolerance is the inability to digest lactose, the sugar found naturally in milk and milk products. Those with lactose intolerance are unable to make enough **lactase,** an enzyme made in the small intestine that helps digest and absorb lactose into the bloodstream.

◄ *SEE ALSO 1.2, "Sugars"* ►

◄ *SEE ALSO 6.7, "Milk"* ►

According to the National Institute of Diabetes and Digestive and Kidney Diseases (NIDDK), an estimated 30–50 million Americans have lactose intolerance. Most people with lactose intolerance have primary lactase deficiency, a condition in which the body's production of lactase is gradually reduced as one gets older. Gastrointestinal diseases such as **celiac disease** or **Crohn's disease** and other conditions that adversely affect small intestine function can cause secondary lactase deficiency, as can bowel surgery and bacterial or viral infection. In some cases, this kind of lactose intolerance can be temporary. Though rare, an infant can be born with congenital lactose intolerance.

◄ *SEE ALSO 9.4, "Gluten Sensitivity"* ►

Others at high risk for lactose intolerance include

> ▶ African Americans, Indian Americans, and Asian Americans
> ▶ Premature infants (because high levels of lactase are produced in late pregnancy)

9.3

Symptoms

When an individual with lactose intolerance consumes lactose, the lactose that's unabsorbed passes through the gastrointestinal tract and into the colon;

bacteria in the colon use that lactose to form hydrogen gas. Symptoms can occur anywhere from 30 minutes to 2 hours after consuming lactose and can include the following:

- Gas
- Bloating
- Stomach cramps or pain
- Nausea
- Diarrhea

Because the symptoms of lactose intolerance can be similar to those that occur as a result of food allergies, other food intolerances, foodborne illnesses, or other conditions or diseases, a physician may perform three tests to diagnose lactose intolerance:

- **Lactose tolerance test**
- **Hydrogen breath test**
- **Stool acidity test**

Unlike those who are allergic to cow's milk and need to avoid all milk products to prevent an allergic reaction, those with lactose intolerance can often consume small amounts of lactose—typically one-half cup, sometimes even as much as a cup—without experiencing symptoms. Age, ethnic background, and other factors determine if and how much lactose an individual can consume without causing symptoms.

◀ *SEE ALSO 9.1, "Food Allergies"* ▶

Dietary Treatment

Although lactose intolerance is not dangerous, several dietary strategies can help individuals with the condition to limit or avoid symptoms.

Lactose is commonly found in dairy foods, such as cow's milk, acidophilus milk, buttermilk, yogurt, cheeses (including American, Swiss, bleu, and Parmesan cheeses), cream, cream cheese, sour cream, ice cream, sherbet, and half-and-half. It can also be found in the following products:

- Bread and other baked goods
- Ready-to-eat breakfast cereals
- Breakfast and meal-replacement beverages
- Instant potatoes and soups
- Non-Kosher lunch meats

▶ Salad dressings

▶ Candies and snack foods

▶ Pancake, brownie, cookie, and muffin mixes

Dietary supplements, over-the-counter antacid and other medications, and birth control pills can also contain lactose.

Reading ingredient lists on foods, beverages, dietary supplements, and prescription medication packages is essential to determine which items contain lactose (although amounts will vary). If any of the following are listed on the ingredients list, the product contains lactose. However, keep in mind that you do not need to avoid all lactose, just large amounts.

INGREDIENTS THAT INDICATE THE PRESENCE OF LACTOSE

Butter	Caseinate	Cheese
Cream	Condensed milk	Curds
Dried milk	Dry milk solids	Evaporated milk
Lactose	Malted milk	Margarine
Milk	Milk byproducts	Milk derivative
Milk solids	Milk sugar	Nonfat dry milk powder (unreconstituted)
Skim milk solids	Whey	Yogurt

◀ *SEE ALSO 10.1, "Reading Food Labels"* ▶

You can experiment with different amounts of lactose-containing foods and beverages, especially nutrient-dense options from the Milk category (including low-fat milk and yogurt). If you know you can't tolerate the amounts of such foods recommended in MyPyramid, be sure to include key nutrients found in milk (including calcium, vitamin D, riboflavin, and protein) from other dietary sources to meet your daily nutrient needs. Alternatively, you can discuss supplements with your physician or a registered dietitian.

◀ *SEE ALSO 3.6, "Daily Protein Recommendations"* ▶

◀ *SEE ALSO 4.8, "Daily Vitamin Recommendations"* ▶

◀ *SEE ALSO 5.9, "Daily Mineral Recommendations"* ▶

◀ *SEE ALSO 10.5, "Dietary Supplements"* ▶

9.3

You can also pair small amounts of lactose-containing foods with foods rich in fiber or protein, which slows digestion, enhancing lactose absorption.

◀ SEE ALSO 1.4, *"Dietary Fiber"* ▶

◀ SEE ALSO 3.3, *"Animal Sources of Protein"* ▶

◀ SEE ALSO 3.4, *"Plant Sources of Protein"* ▶

Although "lactose-free" or "lactose-reduced" milk (such as Lact-Aid) and other dairy products are available, these terms are not officially defined by the FDA. Nevertheless, such products can help you reduce your overall lactose consumption by replacing similar lactose-containing foods and beverages.

Lactase enzymes are also sold as chewable tablets or pills (capsules); you can take these right before you consume lactose-containing foods and beverages to help your body better digest and absorb the lactose and avoid adverse symptoms.

For children or infants with lactose intolerance, calcium-fortified soy milk or rice milk can substitute for cow's milk.

◀ SEE ALSO 9.4, *"Gluten Sensitivity"* ▶

WORDS TO GO . . . WORDS TO GO . . . WORDS TO GO

Lactase is an enzyme (a protein) that breaks down lactose (the sugar in milk and milk products) into glucose and galactose.

Celiac disease is an inherited condition in which gluten—a protein found in grains such as wheat, barley, and rye—cannot be digested.

Crohn's disease is a chronic inflammatory bowel disease that involves the small or large intestine that can cause diarrhea, malabsorption, and other symptoms.

A **lactose tolerance test** is one of several tests used to detect lactose intolerance in adults. It measures the ability of your intestines to break down lactose, the sugar found in milk and other dairy products. Multiple blood tests are taken before and after consuming a lactose-containing solution.

A **hydrogen breath test** is one of several tests used to detect lactose intolerance in adults. It measures how much hydrogen you breathe out and is a noninvasive test commonly used to detect lactose intolerance. Increased hydrogen levels indicate the body is adequately breaking down and absorbing lactose.

A **stool acidity test** is one of several tests used to detect lactose intolerance in children. It measures how acidic a stool sample is after ingesting a small amount of lactose.

9.4   GLUTEN SENSITIVITY

Celiac Disease

Gluten Intolerance

Dietary Treatment for Gluten Sensitivity

In this subchapter, you learn about celiac disease and gluten intolerance. You'll learn how they differ from one another, their causes, and common symptoms associated with each. You also learn about the gluten-free diet, the main treatment for gluten sensitivity.

Celiac Disease

In this section, you learn about celiac disease, including its causes and symptoms.

Definition and Causes

Celiac disease, also known as gluten-sensitive enteropathy, is a chronic digestive disease in which gluten—the main protein found in wheat, rye, and barley damages the lining of the small intestine. When someone with celiac disease consumes gluten-containing foods or beverages, the gluten can't be fully digested and interacts with the immune system of the gastrointestinal tract, triggering an **inflammatory response.** This damages the **villi** of the small intestine (those numerous hair-like extensions that line the inside of the small intestine multiplying exponentially its surface area, so that it can absorb nutrients from digested food as it passes), which causes vitamins, minerals, and other nutrients to pass through the digestive system without being absorbed. This can lead to serious nutrient deficiencies including iron-deficiency anemia or conditions such as **malnutrition** and **osteoporosis.**

◀ SEE ALSO *Chapter 5, "Minerals"* ▶

◀ SEE ALSO *Chapter 8.6, "Osteoporosis"* ▶

Celiac disease increases an individual's risk for other **autoimmune conditions** such as type 1 diabetes, rheumatoid arthritis, or thyroid problems. It can also increase the risk for some gastrointestinal cancers.

◀ SEE ALSO *8.3, "Diabetes"* ▶

◀ SEE ALSO *8.5, "Cancer"* ▶

9.4

Celiac disease is one of the most common inherited diseases and affects about 1 percent of the U.S. population. Although anyone can develop the condition, those at high risk include

▶ Those with a first-degree relative (such as a parent) who has celiac disease

▶ Those of Northern European decent

▶ Those who have a genetic disorder such as **Down's syndrome** or **Turner syndrome**

Adults (especially older ones) are diagnosed more often then children, and the prevalence of celiac disease is greater in women than in men. Diagnosis often occurs 10 or more years after the condition develops, in part because there can be few or no symptoms. Sometimes, it is diagnosed for the first time after surgery, pregnancy, childbirth, a viral infection, or severe emotional stress, or when an individual seeks medical care for another condition.

Although genes play a big role in determining who develops celiac disease and when, there's some evidence that breastfeeding while introducing gluten-containing foods, or gradually introducing gluten-containing foods into an infant's diet between 4 and 6 months of age (not earlier or later) can reduce the risk of developing celiac disease in early childhood and possibly later in life as well.

Symptoms

Although some individuals with celiac disease might not experience symptoms, others might. A person's age and whether he has any other diseases or conditions can affect whether he has symptoms or the types exhibited. Symptoms can include some of the following:

▶ Diarrhea

▶ Constipation

▶ Abdominal pain, bloating, or gas

▶ Nausea

▶ Vomiting

▶ **Reduced gut motility**

▶ Delayed gastric emptying

▶ Weakness

▶ Unintentional weight loss

▶ **Failure to thrive** in infants

▶ Short stature or delayed puberty

About 10–20 percent of those with celiac disease have **dermatitis herpetiformis,** a chronic skin rash. Chronic fatigue, infertility or miscarriage, neurological problems (including seizures and difficulties with memory or concentration), muscle cramps, and migraine headaches can also occur more frequently in those with celiac disease.

Diagnosing celiac disease can be difficult, especially in young children. A physician can use family history and symptoms as initial screening tools, followed by blood tests that check for the presence of antibodies (such as IgA and IgG anti-endomysial antibodies [AEMAs]) or for the autoantigen, a substance that triggers the altered immune response seen in celiac disease (IgA and IgG antitissue transglutaminase [ATTGA]). A biopsy of the small intestine is recommended for those whose blood test results are positive. If the biopsy is also positive, and if the individual improves by following a gluten-free diet, this confirms the diagnosis of celiac disease.

Gluten Intolerance

In this section, you learn about gluten intolerance, including its causes and symptoms.

Definition and Causes

Like celiac disease, gluten intolerance is a condition in which ingesting gluten, the main protein in wheat, rye, and barley, causes an adverse reaction in the body. The body's innate immune system recognizes gluten as an enemy and immediately works to eliminate it from the body. However, ingesting gluten does not cause intestinal villi damage or other permanent organ damage in gluten intolerance the way it does in celiac disease.

Symptoms

Although gluten sensitivity is not a food allergy, nor does it cause an autoimmune response (as seen in celiac disease), it can cause similar symptoms including abdominal pain and bloating, diarrhea, and fatigue. Joint pain and reflux can also occur. Although no specific tests are used to diagnose gluten intolerance, some experts recommend testing for both wheat allergy and celiac disease if gluten sensitivity is suspected. If tests for these conditions are negative, the person with symptoms should try eliminating gluten-containing foods from

9.4

the diet and then, under the supervision of a doctor or a registered dietitian, reintroduce them to see if and how that affects symptoms.

Dietary Treatment for Gluten Sensitivity

There is no cure for celiac disease or gluten intolerance; avoiding gluten for life is recommended to reduce or resolve symptoms and some of the health and nutritional problems associated with celiac disease and gluten intolerance. Starting a gluten-free diet is not advised before a firm diagnosis is made, however, because doing so can decrease the accuracy of the test results.

Those diagnosed with celiac disease or gluten intolerance should consult with a registered dietitian to learn how to avoid gluten while consuming adequate calories and nutrients to meet individual needs. You can find a registered dietitian in your area by contacting the American Dietetic Association at www.eatright.org.

Gluten-Free Diet

Gluten is found in wheat, rye, barley, and the variety of foods and beverages made with them, including many kinds of breads, baked goods, cereals, pastas, bouillon cubes, soups, sauces (soy sauce and gravy), seasonings, salad dressings, snack foods (such as potato or tortilla chips), prepared meats (deli meats, hot dogs, hamburger patties, and imitation seafood), imitation fish, egg substitutes, French fries, vegetables in sauce, yogurt drinks, frozen yogurt, flavored coffees and teas, and some candies (such as licorice and chocolate bars). Some dietary supplements and medications can also contain gluten, as does the glue found on envelopes and stamps.

Oat, corn, and rice products do not contain gluten themselves, but often become contaminated when made in factories that also manufacture wheat products.

Reading food labels (ingredient lists in particular) is critical for those with celiac disease. Although wheat is a "major food allergen" listed on ingredients lists on food packages, you'll need to be savvy to identify other sources of gluten.

◄ SEE ALSO 9.1, *"Food Allergies"* ►

◄ SEE ALSO 10.1, *"Reading Food Labels"* ►

The following table lists gluten-containing foods and ingredients to avoid when following a gluten-free diet:

GLUTEN-CONTAINING FOODS AND INGREDIENTS TO AVOID

Wheat

Atta*	Matzoh, Matzoh meal
Bulgur	Kamut**
Couscous	Modified wheat starch
Dinkel (also known as spelt)	Seitan****
Durum**	Semolina
Einkorn**	Spelt (also known as farro or faro; dinkel)
Farina	Triticale
Farro or faro (also known as spelt)**	Wheat bran
Fu***	Wheat flour
Graham flour	Wheat germ
Hydrolyzed wheat protein	Wheat starch

*A fine whole-meal flour made from low-gluten, soft-textured wheat used to make Indian flatbread (known as chapatti flour).

**Types of wheat.

***A dried gluten product derived from wheat that is sold as thin sheets or thick round cakes. Used as a protein supplement in Asian dishes such as soups and vegetables.

****A meat-like food derived from wheat gluten used in many vegetarian dishes. Sometimes called "wheat meat."

Barley

Ale*	Malt extract
Barley (flakes, flour, pearl)	Malt syrup
Beer*	Malt flavoring***
Brewer's yeast	Malt vinegar
Lager*	Malted milk
Malt**	

*Most regular ale, beer, and lager are derived from barley, which is not gluten-free. However, there are several new varieties of gluten-free beer derived from buckwheat, sorghum, and/or rice, which are gluten-free.

**Malt is an enzyme preparation usually derived from sprouted barley, which is not gluten-free. Other cereal grains can also be malted and might or might not be gluten-free depending on the additional ingredients used in the malting process.

***These terms are used interchangeably to denote a concentrated liquid solution of barley malt that is used as a flavoring agent.

Rye

Rye bread	Rye flour

continues

9.4

GLUTEN-CONTAINING FOODS AND INGREDIENTS TO AVOID (CONTINUED)

Oats*

Oatmeal	Oat flour
Oat bran	Oats

Celiac organizations in Canada and the United States do not recommend consumption of commercially available oat products because they are often cross-contaminated with wheat or barley. However, pure, uncontaminated specialty gluten-free oat products from North America are now available, and many organizations allow consumption of moderate amounts of these oats for persons with celiac disease.

Source: Shelley Case, BSc, RD, Gluten-Free Diet: A Comprehensive Resource Guide, *2008.*

Here are some gluten-free flours, cereals, and starches that people with gluten sensitivity can safely consume (courtesy of Shelley Case, BSc, RD's *Gluten-Free Diet: A Comprehensive Resource Guide* [2008]):

Gluten-Free Flours, Cereals, and Starches

▶ Amaranth

▶ Arrowroot

▶ Buckwheat

▶ Corn

▶ Flax

▶ Indian ricegrass (Montina)

▶ Legume flours (bean, chickpea/garbanzo, lentil, pea)

▶ Mesquite flour

▶ Millet

▶ Nut flours (almond, hazelnut, pecan)

▶ Potato flour

▶ Potato starch

▶ Quinoa

▶ Rice (black, brown, glutinous/sweet, white, wild)

▶ Rice bran

▶ Rice polish

▶ Sago

▶ Sorghum

▶ Soy

▶ Sweet potato flour

▶ Tapioca (cassava/manioc)

▶ Teff

Although some studies have shown that consuming pure oats (about 50 grams a day, or the amount in ½ cup rolled oats) can be safe and help those with celiac disease comply with a gluten-free diet, there is controversy over whether oats can contribute to gastrointestinal and other symptoms. Many experts believe that oats often produce symptoms because of contamination with wheat during processing. So look for brands that guarantee their oats are gluten-free.

The FDA recently proposed a definition of the term "gluten-free" that manufacturers can use voluntarily on food packages. According to the FDA's proposed definition, a product labeled "gluten-free" does not contain

▶ An ingredient that is a "prohibited grain." This includes any species of wheat (such as durum wheat, spelt wheat, and Kamut), rye, barley, or their crossbred hybrids.

▶ An ingredient (such as wheat flour) derived from a "prohibited grain" that has not been processed to remove gluten.

▶ An ingredient (such as wheat starch) that is derived from a "prohibited grain" that has been processed to remove gluten, if the use of that ingredient results in the presence of ≥ 20 micrograms of gluten per food.

▶ ≥ 20 micrograms of gluten per gram of food.

If a food product says "no gluten," "without gluten," "free of gluten" and doesn't meet the previously specified conditions, the FDA will consider that item misbranded.

◀ *SEE ALSO 10.1, "Reading Food Labels"* ▶

The Gluten Intolerance Group developed a voluntary, independent food processing inspection program called the Gluten Free Certification Organization in August 2005 to test and monitor ingredients in, and the processing of, gluten-free products. It allows qualified foods to put a "gluten-free" certification mark on their package. To qualify, a food must contain < 10 ppm gluten (or 3 milligrams).

People with celiac disease can malabsorb nutrients such as iron, calcium, folate, carbohydrates, fat, and fat-soluble vitamins (A, D, E, and K) so they may require nutrient supplementation. This should be discussed with a physician or registered dietitian.

◀ *SEE ALSO 1.5, "Daily Carbohydrate Recommendations"* ▶

◀ *SEE ALSO 2.7, "Daily Fat and Cholesterol Recommendations"* ▶

◀ *SEE ALSO Chapter 4, "Vitamins"* ▶

9.4

◀ *SEE ALSO Chapter 5, "Minerals"* ▶

◀ *SEE ALSO 10.5, "Dietary Supplements"* ▶

WORDS TO GO . . .WORDS TO GO . . .WORDS TO GO

An **inflammatory response** refers to a reaction by the body characterized by the release of cells and chemicals to repair damage caused by disease or injury.

Villi are tiny fingerlike protrusions that line the small intestine and help nutrients from food get absorbed into the bloodstream.

Malnutrition is a condition that develops when the body doesn't receive enough vitamins, minerals, and other nutrients required to meet its needs and maintain healthy tissues and organ function.

Osteoporosis is a condition in which bones become porous because they've lost too much protein and minerals such as calcium. This leads to reduced bone mass and bone strength and increases the risk of fracture.

An **autoimmune condition** is one in which the body wages an immune response against one of its own tissues, cells, or molecules.

Down's syndrome is the most common cause of mental retardation and malformation in a newborn. It is caused by the presence of an extra chromosome (structures in the nucleus of every cell in the body that contain the genetic information necessary for growth and normal body functions).

Turner syndrome is a chromosomal disorder that affects females. In this condition, one of the two x chromosomes is damaged or nonexistent. This leads to impaired growth (with lack of a growth spurt in puberty), small stature, and frequent infertility.

Reduced gut motility is slower movement of food through the small intestine. This can contribute to constipation and other gastrointestinal problems.

Failure to thrive is a cluster of symptoms characterized by delayed growth or development in infants and children up to age 2.

Dermatitis herpetiformis is a rare, chronic, autoimmune skin disorder associated with celiac disease that's characterized by itchy, blistering skin; it most often affects skin on the knees, back, elbows, and buttocks.

Definition and Causes
Symptoms
Who Is at Risk

This subchapter provides a broad overview of food poisoning, including its causes, its symptoms, and who is most at risk. In Chapter 12, specific organisms and other substances in food that cause foodborne illnesses are reviewed in greater detail.

Definition and Causes

Food poisoning, more accurately called **foodborne illness,** is classified as a **food intolerance.** It occurs after consuming contaminated foods or beverages. In most cases, foodborne illnesses are caused by **microorganisms** or **microbes** such as bacteria, viruses, and parasites, although natural toxins and chemicals found in foods can also cause food-related sickness.

◄ *SEE ALSO 12.1 "Foodborne Pathogens"* ►

◄ *SEE ALSO 12.2, "Other Harmful Substances in Food"* ►

Most people who develop foodborne illnesses don't report them, perhaps because they don't realize their symptoms came from something they ate or drank. The Centers for Disease Control (CDC) estimates that 76 million cases of foodborne diseases occur each year in the United States.

Although any food or beverage can become contaminated, some of the usual suspects include the following: animal proteins, moist foods, and raw produce.

Protein-rich animal foods, including meat, poultry, fish, and seafood (especially when consumed raw or undercooked), are often involved in outbreaks of foodborne illness. During processing, animals' intestinal contents, which harbor microorganisms, can come into contact with carcasses and contaminate them. Also, the protein found in animal foods is broken down into amino acids; some bacteria use these as a nutrient source.

◄ *SEE ALSO 3.3, "Animal Sources of Protein"* ►

9.5

Moist foods that are creamy or made with eggs (including potato and pasta salads, cream-based soups, and custard or cream pies) provide an environment in which bacteria thrive and multiply. Contrary to popular opinion, however, mayonnaise does not make a food more risky; in fact, it's just the opposite. The acidity of mayonnaise helps protect from bacterial growth.

Fruits and vegetables such as spinach, lettuce, tomatoes, sprouts, and melons and other produce can cause foodborne illness if contaminated when grown, harvested, processed, stored, or otherwise handled. It's not uncommon for produce to cause illness when it's washed with water that has been contaminated by human sewage or animal manure. Because many of these foods are eaten raw, there is no chance to kill the microorganisms if present. Thorough washing is your only defense.

Symptoms

Usually, foodborne illnesses that strike otherwise healthy people cause mild symptoms, including diarrhea, nausea, stomach cramps, and fever.

The types, onset, and duration of symptoms of foodborne illness vary depending on the cause of the illness and other factors. In most cases, symptoms occur within several hours or a few days, but symptoms can occur weeks or even months after exposure to a disease-causing microorganism. Some symptoms are mild and last several hours to a few days, whereas others are more severe and last for weeks or even months. And sometimes, consuming tainted foods or beverages can cause other severe infections and, in some cases, even death. The CDC estimates that foodborne illnesses are responsible for 325,000 hospitalizations and 5,000 deaths in the United States each year.

◀ *SEE ALSO Chapter 12, "Foodborne Illnesses and Food Safety"* ▶

Who Is at Risk

Although anyone can develop foodborne illnesses, some segments of the population are more susceptible and can suffer more pronounced or severe consequences from them. Often, their age or stage of life, a medical condition, or their health status has resulted in a weakened or underdeveloped immune system that impairs their ability to fight off harmful **pathogens.** Those at greatest risk for foodborne illnesses include

- ▶ Infants and young children
- ▶ Older people
- ▶ Pregnant women and their unborn fetuses

▶ Those with HIV infection

▶ Those with diabetes or cancer

◀ *SEE ALSO 8.3, "Diabetes"* ▷

◀ *SEE ALSO 8.5, "Cancer"* ▷

▶ Those on steroid therapy for asthma, arthritis, or other conditions

▶ Those with alcoholism

▶ Those with liver or kidney disease

▶ Those with **hemochromatosis**

▶ Those with stomach problems (including low stomach acid because of chronic antacid use or a history of stomach surgery)

WORDS TO GO . . . *WORDS TO GO . . . WORDS TO GO*

Foodborne illness is an infectious or toxic disease that occurs after consuming contaminated food.

A **food intolerance** is a reaction to food that involves the digestive system but not the immune system (as in a true food allergy). It occurs when a food component irritates the digestive system or when it cannot be properly digested or broken down in the body.

Microorganisms or **microbes** are extremely small organisms such as bacteria and fungi.

Pathogens are microorganisms including viruses, bacteria, and fungi that contribute to the development of disease.

Hemochromatosis is an inherited blood disorder that causes the body to retain excess amounts of the mineral iron; over time, a buildup of iron in the body can cause conditions including heart failure, liver cancer, or cirrhosis of the liver. It is more likely to cause serious problems in men and is easily detected through blood tests

9.5

10

HEALTHY FOOD SHOPPING

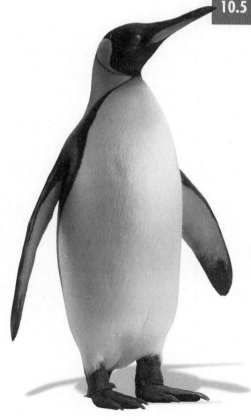

10.1 READING FOOD LABELS

Overview

Nutrition Facts Panel

Ingredients List

In this subchapter, you are introduced to food labels. You learn how to read nutrition facts panels and ingredients on food products to help you make more informed and healthful selections when shopping for food.

Overview

Food labels have been required on most processed and packaged foods since the passage of the Federal Food, Drug, and Cosmetic Act in 1906; it was not until 1973 that voluntary nutrient labeling of food products began. In 1990, the Nutrition Labeling and Education Act (NLEA) led to the development of the nutrition facts panel, required on food labels since 1994.

Food labels provide consumers with information to help them make more informed, healthful choices when shopping for food. By law, food labels are required to contain the following:

- ▶ **A statement of identity**
- ▶ The **net contents** of the package
- ▶ The name and address of the manufacturer, packer, or distributor
- ▶ An ingredients list
- ▶ Nutrition information

Nutrition Facts Panel

A nutrition facts panel appears on virtually all packaged food labels. It provides valuable information to help consumers make more informed and healthful selections when shopping for groceries.

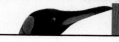

What a food label contains.

(Courtesy of the Food and Drug Administration's Center for Food Safety and Applied Nutrition; www.cfsan.fda.gov/~dms/label-dl.html)

Nutrition Facts

Serving Size 1 cup (228g)
Servings Per Container 2

Amount Per Serving	
Calories 250	Calories from Fat 110

	% Daily Value*
Total Fat 12g	**18%**
Saturated Fat 3g	**15%**
Trans Fat 1.5g	
Cholesterol 30mg	**10%**
Sodium 470mg	**20%**
Total Carbohydrate 31g	**10%**
Dietary Fiber 0g	**0%**
Sugars 5g	
Protein 5g	

Vitamin A	4%
Vitamin C	2%
Calcium	20%
Iron	4%

* Percent Daily Values are based on a 2,000 calorie diet. Your Daily Values may be higher or lower depending on your calorie needs:

	Calories:	2,000	2,500
Total Fat	Less than	65g	80g
Sat Fat	Less than	20g	25g
Cholesterol	Less than	300mg	300mg
Sodium	Less than	2,400mg	2,400mg
Total Carbohydrate		300g	375g
Dietary Fiber		25g	30g

Found on the side or back of a food package, the nutrition facts panel contains the following information:

▶ Serving size—This reflects the amount of food the government considers to be a typical serving size. Within some categories, serving sizes for different products may not be the same, so it's important to consider this when comparing products. For example, one serving of one ready-to-eat cereal might be ¾ cup, whereas one serving of another might be 1½ cups. Servings per container tells you how many servings are in the entire package.

▶ Calories—This is a measure of the amount of energy in one serving of the item. The number of servings you consume determines how many calories you derive from the product. For example, if a cereal has 110 calories for a 1-cup serving but you eat 2 cups, that's 110 × 2 = 220 calories.

10.1

▶ Calories from fat—This is useful because of all the key macronutrients (carbohydrates, fat, and protein), fat provides the most calories per gram. Being aware of the amount of fat you consume and cutting back on total fat intake can likely help you curb your total calorie intake.

◀ SEE ALSO 2.7, *"Daily Fat and Cholesterol Recommendations"* ▶

▶ Nutrients of concern—The following five nutrients appear on labels and tend to be those Americans often don't get enough of and should increase in the diet):

1. Fiber

2. Vitamin A

3. Vitamin C

4. Calcium

5. Iron

◀ SEE ALSO Chapter 4, *"Vitamins"* ▶

◀ SEE ALSO Chapter 5, *"Minerals"* ▶

▶ Other specific nutrients—The following nutrients also appear on food labels. With the exception of protein, these nutrients are those Americans tend to overconsume and should decrease in the diet; They include

▶ Saturated fat (listed under total fat)

▶ Trans fat (listed under total fat)

▶ Cholesterol

▶ Sodium

▶ Protein

◀ SEE ALSO Chapter 3, *"Proteins"* ▶

◀ SEE ALSO Chapter 11, *"Healthy Eating Habits"* ▶

▶ Sugar is listed under total carbohydrate. The nutrition facts panel does not yet distinguish between sugar that's naturally occurring (such as lactose in milk and fructose in fruit) and sugar that's added to food. Because Americans tend to overconsume added sugar, current dietary guidelines recommend decreasing added sugar intake. Ingredients lists on food labels (which will be discussed later) can help consumers identify added sugars found in products.

◄ *SEE ALSO 6.9, "Discretionary Calories"* ▣

◄ *SEE ALSO Chapter 3, "Proteins"* ▣

▶ Percent Daily Value—Daily Value (DV) is a dietary reference value based on Daily Reference Values (DRVs) and Reference Daily Intakes (RDIs) that helps Americans compare nutrients found in different foods. It is based on a standard 2,000-calorie diet. A food that contains 10–19 percent of the DV for a nutrient is a "good source" of that nutrient; one that boasts at least 20 percent of the DV for a nutrient is "high" in, or a rich source of, that nutrient. Here are the daily values for various nutrients:

REFERENCE VALUES FOR NUTRITION LABELING*

Nutrient	Daily Value (DV)
Total fat	65 grams
Saturated fat	20 grams
Cholesterol	300 milligrams
Sodium	2,400 milligrams
Potassium	3,500 milligrams
Total carbohydrate	300 grams
Fiber	25 grams
Protein	50 grams
Vitamin A	5,000 international units (IUs)
Vitamin C	60 milligrams
Calcium	1,000 milligrams
Iron	18 milligrams
Vitamin D	400 IUs
Vitamin E	30 IUs
Vitamin K	80 micrograms
Thiamin	1.5 milligrams
Riboflavin	1.7 milligrams
Niacin	20 milligrams
Vitamin B6	2.0 milligrams
Folate	400 micrograms
Vitamin B12	6.0 micrograms
Biotin	300 micrograms
Pantothenic acid	10 milligrams
Phosphorus	1,000 milligrams

10.1

continues

REFERENCE VALUES FOR NUTRITION LABELING* (CONTINUED)

Nutrient	Daily Value (DV)
Iodine	150 micrograms
Magnesium	400 milligrams
Zinc	15 milligrams
Selenium	70 micrograms
Copper	2.0 milligrams
Manganese	2.0 milligrams
Chromium	120 micrograms
Molybdenum	75 micrograms
Chloride	3,400 milligrams

*Based on a 2,000-calorie diet; for adults and children ages 4 and above; this list includes only those nutrients for which a DRV or a RDI has been established.

Source: Food and Drug Administration.

Some nutrients can be voluntarily included on nutrition facts panels. This includes calories from saturated fat; polyunsaturated fat; potassium, soluble, and insoluble fiber; sugar alcohols; **other carbohydrates;** other vitamins and minerals; and percent of vitamin A present as beta-carotene.

Ingredients List

On food labels, ingredients are listed by their common or usual names in descending order by weight. Those that appear first are the most prominent, while those listed last are the least prominent. The following must also be included on ingredients lists:

- ▶ Any of the "8 Major Allergens"
- ▶ FDA-certified color additives
- ▶ Specific ingredient information (for example, the source of the protein)

◀ SEE ALSO 9.1, *"Food Allergies"* ▶

A warning statement must be provided on food packages of items that contain food additives such as aspartame (an artificial sweetener) and sulfites (a preservative) that can potentially be harmful if consumed by certain people.

◀ SEE ALSO 9.2, *"Food Additive Sensitivities"* ▶

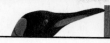

Also, when a preservative or some other additive is used in a product, it must be listed by its common name and its function (the terms "preservative," "to retard spoilage," "a mold inhibitor," "to help protect flavor," or "to promote color retention") can be used.

WORDS TO GO . . .WORDS TO GO . . .WORDS TO GO

A **statement of identity** is a mandate that commercial food products display prominently the common or usual name of the product or identify the food with an "appropriately descriptive term."

Net contents refers to the weight, volume, measure, or numerical amount of food contained in the package.

Other carbohydrates, when listed on a nutrition facts panel, refers to the difference between total carbohydrate and the sum of dietary fiber, sugars, and sugar alcohol.

10.1

10.2 UNDERSTANDING CLAIMS ON FOOD PACKAGES

Nutrient Content Claims

Health Claims

Qualified Health Claims

Structure/Function Claims

Dietary Guidance Statements

This subchapter provides an overview and examples of nutrient content, health, and structure/function claims that appear on packaged foods and in dietary supplements.

Nutrient Content Claims

A nutrient content claim (NCC), often found on the front of a food package, indicates the amount of a nutrient a product contains. The Nutrition Labeling and Education Act (NLEA) and FDA have created definitions for and allowed use of terms including "low-fat," "sodium free," and "good source" on food packages as a tool to help consumers make more healthful food selections based on their individual needs and preferences. Here are standard definitions for NNCs often found on food packages:

NUTRIENT CONTENT CLAIMS ON FOOD LABELS

Term	Definition
Calorie free	Less than 5 calories per serving.
Cholesterol free	Less than 2 mg* cholesterol and 2 grams or less saturated fat per serving.
Enriched or fortified	Has been nutritionally altered so that one serving provides at least 10 percent more of the DV of a nutrient than the comparison food.
Extra lean	Less than 5 grams fat, 2 grams saturated fat, and 95 mg* of cholesterol per serving and per 100 grams.
Fat-free	Less than 0.5 grams of fat per serving.
Free	"Without, "No," or "Zero" can all be used in place of "free"**.

Term	Definition
Fresh	Generally used on food in its raw state; cannot be used on a food that has been frozen or cooked or on food that contains preservatives.
Fresh-frozen	Foods that have been quickly frozen while still fresh.
Good source	One serving provides 10–19 percent of the daily value for a particular nutrient.
Good source of fiber	The DV for fiber (2.5–4.75 grams) per serving; if a food is not "low-fat," it must declare the level of total fat per serving and refer to the nutrition panel when a fiber claim is made.
High	One serving provides 20 percent or more of the DV for a particular nutrient.
High fiber	Contains 20 percent or more of the DV for fiber (at least 5 grams) per serving; if a food is not "low-fat," it must declare level of total fat per serving and refer to the nutrition panel when a fiber claim is made.
Lean	Less than 10 grams of fat, 4 grams of saturated fat, and 95 mg* of cholesterol per serving and per 100 grams.
Light	1) At least ⅓ fewer calories per serving than a comparison food, or 2) Contains no more than half the fat per serving of a comparison food; if a food derives 50 percent or more of its calories from fat, the reduction must be at least 50 percent of the fat; 3) Contains at least 50 percent less sodium per serving than a comparison food; or 4) Can refer to texture and/or color, if clearly explained, for example "light brown sugar."
Low	"Little," "few," or "low source of" may be used in place of "low."
Low calorie	40 calories or less per serving.
Low cholesterol	20 milligrams or less cholesterol and 2 grams or less of saturated fat per serving.
Low fat	3 grams or less per serving.

continues

10.2

NUTRIENT CONTENT CLAIMS ON FOOD LABELS (CONTINUED)

Term	Definition
Low saturated fat	1 gram or less per serving and 15 percent or less calories from fat.
Low sodium	140 mg* or less per serving.
More	One serving contains at least 10 percent or more of the DV of a nutrient than a comparison food.
Percent fat free	A claim made on a "low fat" or "fat free" product that accurately reflects the amount of fat present in 100 grams of food; a food with 3 grams of fat per 100 grams would be "97 percent fat free."
Reduced	A nutritionally altered product that must contain 25 percent less of a nutrient or of calories than the regular or reference product.
Salt or sodium free	Less than 5 mg* per serving.
Sugar free	Less than 0.5 grams of sugars per serving.
Unsalted	Has no salt added during processing; to use this term, the product it resembles must normally be processed with salt and the label must note that the food is not a sodium-free food if it does not meet the requirements for "sodium" free.
Very low sodium	35 mg* or less sodium per serving.

mg = milligrams

**For example, a "calorie-free" or "fat-free" food can also say "zero calories" or "zero fat."*

Source: Understanding the Food Label, Colorado State University Cooperative Extension, www.ext.colostate.edu.

A **disclosure statement** must be made on products that contain an NCC if they contain nutrients in the following amounts (per serving or per 50 grams, or 2 ounces of the product if it comes in a small package) because these amounts can increase the risk of a diet-related disease or condition:

▶ Total fat—Greater than 13 grams

▶ Saturated fat—Greater than 4 grams

▶ Cholesterol—Greater than 60 milligrams

▶ Sodium—Greater than 480 milligrams

A meal-type product (a product that weighs between 6 and 12 ounces per serving and contains ingredients from two or more of four specified food groups) needs a disclosure statement if, per labeled serving, it contains more than 26 grams of fat, 8 grams of saturated fat, 120 milligrams of cholesterol, or 960 milligrams of sodium. Similarly, a main dish product (a product that weighs at least 6 ounces and contains at least two different foods from at least two of four specified food groups) must bear a disclosure statement if it contains (per labeled serving) more than 19.5 grams of fat, 6.0 grams of saturated fat, 90 milligrams of cholesterol, or 720 milligrams of sodium.

A manufacturer can also make a claim about a nutrient that has no established DV as long as it simply states the amount of that nutrient per labeled serving (and not the level of the nutrient in the product). For example, "x grams of omega-3 fatty acids" can be made and placed somewhere on the food package (but not on the nutrition facts panel).

Health Claims

Health claims are statements on food packages that associate a particular food (or substance or nutrient in that food) with a reduction in a diet-related disease or condition (but not the treatment, diagnosis, cure, or mitigation of a disease or condition). Health claims must be supported by scientifically valid evidence and must include an amount of the particular nutrient or food that is directly associated with the diet-related disease or condition.

The FDA reviews and evaluates all health claims and authorizes their use on food packages only if there is "significant scientific agreement" supporting the particular health claim. Thus far, the following health claims have been approved by the FDA (an example of how that claim may be stated on a food package is provided for each):

> ▶ Calcium and osteoporosis—Adequate calcium and regular exercise may reduce the risk of osteoporosis.

◀ *SEE ALSO 5.5, "Calcium"* ▶

◀ *SEE ALSO 8.6, "Osteoporosis"* ▶

> ▶ Sodium and hypertension—Low-sodium diets may reduce the risk of hypertension.

◀ *SEE ALSO 5.2, "Sodium"* ▶

◀ *SEE ALSO 8.2, "Hypertension"* ▶

10.2

◀ *SEE ALSO 11.6, "Decreasing Sodium Intake"* ▶

   ▶ Dietary fat and cancer—A diet low in total fat may reduce the risk of some cancers.

◀ *SEE ALSO 2.7, "Daily Fat and Cholesterol Recommendations"* ▶

   ▶ Dietary saturated fat and cholesterol and risk of coronary heart disease— Diets low in saturated fat and cholesterol may reduce the risk of coronary heart disease.

◀ *SEE ALSO 11.3, "Decreasing Saturated Fat Intake"* ▶

◀ *SEE ALSO 11.5, "Decreasing Dietary Cholesterol Intake"* ▶

   ▶ Fiber-containing grain products, fruits, and vegetables and cancer— Low-fat diets rich in fiber-containing grain products, fruits, and vegetables may reduce the risk of some types of cancer.

   ▶ Fruits, vegetables, and grain products that contain fiber, particularly soluble fiber, and risk of coronary heart disease—Diets low in saturated fat and cholesterol and rich in fruits, vegetables, and grain products that contain some types of dietary fiber, particularly soluble fiber, may reduce the risk of heart disease.

   ▶ Fruits and vegetables and cancer—Low-fat diets rich in fruits and vegetables (foods that are low in fat and may contain dietary fiber, vitamin A, or vitamin C) may reduce the risk of some types of cancer.

◀ *SEE ALSO 6.3, "Fruits"* ▶

◀ *SEE ALSO 6.4, "Vegetables"* ▶

◀ *SEE ALSO 8.5, "Cancer"* ▶

   ▶ Folate and neural tube defects—Healthful diets with adequate folate may reduce a woman's risk of having a child with a brain or spinal cord defect.

◀ *SEE ALSO 4.7, "B Vitamins"* ▶

   ▶ Sugar alcohols and dental caries—Frequent between-meal consumption of foods high in sugars and starches promotes tooth decay. The sugar alcohols in [name of food] do not promote tooth decay. (Small packages can simply state "Does not promote tooth decay.")

   ▶ Soluble fiber from certain foods and risk of coronary heart disease— Soluble fiber from [name of fiber source and, if desired, food product], as part of a diet low in saturated fat and cholesterol, may reduce the risk of heart disease. A serving of [name of food product] supplies [x grams] of the [necessary daily dietary intake for the benefit] soluble fiber from [name of soluble fiber source] necessary per day to have this effect.

◁ *SEE ALSO 11.1, "Increasing Fiber Intake"* ▷

▶ Foods that contain fiber from psyllium and risk of heart disease—Diets low in saturated fat and cholesterol that include soluble fiber from psyllium seed husk may reduce the risk of heart disease.

◁ *SEE ALSO 1.4, "Dietary Fiber"* ▷

◁ *SEE ALSO 8.1, "Cardiovascular Disease"* ▷

▶ Soy protein and risk of coronary heart disease—25 grams of soy protein a day, as part of a diet low in saturated fat and cholesterol, may reduce the risk of heart disease. A serving of [name of food] supplies [x grams] of soy protein. Diets low in saturated fat and cholesterol that include 25 grams of soy protein a day may reduce the risk of heart disease. One serving of [name of food] provides [x grams] of soy protein.

◁ *SEE ALSO 3.4, "Plant Sources of Protein"* ▷

◁ *SEE ALSO 6.6, "Meat and Beans"* ▷

◁ *SEE ALSO 8.1, "Cardiovascular Disease"* ▷

▶ Plant sterol/stanol esters and risk of coronary heart disease—Foods containing at least 0.65 gram per of vegetable oil sterol esters, eaten twice a day with meals for a daily total intake of at least 1.3 grams, as part of a diet low in saturated fat and cholesterol may reduce the risk of heart disease. A serving of [name of food] supplies [x grams] of vegetable oil sterol esters. Diets low in saturated fat and cholesterol that include two servings of foods that provide a daily total of at least 3.4 grams of plant stanol esters in two meals can reduce the risk of heart disease. A serving of [name of food] supplies [x grams] of plant stanol esters.

◁ *SEE ALSO 10.3, "Functional Foods"* ▷

Some health claims are authorized based on an authoritative statement by the FDA's Modernization Act (FDAMA) health claims. These include the following:

▶ Whole grain foods and risk of heart disease and certain cancers—Diets rich in whole grain foods and other plant foods and that are low in total fat, saturated fat, and cholesterol may reduce the risk of heart disease and some cancers.

▶ Potassium and the risk of high blood pressure and stroke—Diets containing foods that are a good source of potassium and that are also low in sodium may reduce the risk of high blood pressure and stroke.

▶ Fluoridated water and reduced risk of dental caries—Drinking fluoridated water may reduce the risk of dental caries or tooth decay.

10.2

Qualified Health Claims

Qualified health claims (QHCs) can be made for conventional foods as well as dietary supplements. Although there is some scientific support for these claims, they have not yet reached "significant scientific agreement." Here's an example of what a QHC on a food package can look like:

▶ Scientific evidence suggests but does not prove that eating 1½ ounces of nuts as part of a diet low in saturated fat and cholesterol can reduce risk of heart disease. [See nutrition information for fat content.]

▶ Supportive but not conclusive research shows that consumption of EPA and DHA omega-3 fatty acids may reduce the risk of coronary heart disease. One serving of [name of the food] provides [x grams] of EPA and DHA omega-3 fatty acids.

◀ SEE ALSO 8.1, *"Cardiovascular Disease"* ▶

Structure/Function Claims

Structure/function claims describe the effect of a food or food component on body structures or functions without making reference to a disease. Here are a few examples of structure/function claims:

▶ "...helps promote immune health"

▶ "...is an energizer"

▶ "Calcium builds strong bones"

▶ "Fiber maintains bowel regularity"

Structure/function claims do not need FDA review or approval, but if used, they must be truthful and not misleading.

◀ SEE ALSO 10.5, *"Dietary Supplements"* ▶

Dietary Guidance Statements

Although they're not considered health claims, **dietary guidance statements** that are scientifically sound and not misleading can appear on food packages. These types of statements refer to broad classes of foods (rather than a specific food or substance referred to in health claims) and have scientific support. Here are two examples of a dietary guidance statement:

▶ "Consuming at least 3 or more ounce-equivalents of whole grains per day can reduce the risk of several chronic diseases"

▶ "Carrots are good for your health"

▶ "Calcium is good for you"

Although dietary guidance statements can appear on food packages without FDA approval, they may be reviewed by the FDA at a later point to ensure they're truthful and not misleading.

WORDS TO GO . . . WORDS TO GO . . . WORDS TO GO

A **disclosure statement** is a statement that calls the consumer's attention to one or more nutrients in the food that may increase the risk of a disease or health-related condition that is diet related; it's required when a nutrient in a food exceeds certain prescribed levels.

Dietary guidance statements are statements made on food packages that either associate a class of foods (such as whole grains) to a diet-related disease or condition or refer to a specific food or food component without referring to a disease or health-related condition. They are not health claims and are not subject to approval by the FDA before they can be used.

10.2

10.3 FUNCTIONAL FOODS

Overview

Functional Components in Foods

This subchapter defines functional foods. It also provides examples of the many functional ingredients found naturally in or added to foods that can possibly benefit consumers.

Overview

Functional foods provide health benefits beyond the scope of basic nutrition. Examples include foods that naturally contain healthful substances (such as garlic, which contains sulfur compounds that may reduce the risk of some cancers, and tomatoes, which contain lycopene, an antioxidant shown to reduce prostate cancer risk). Functional foods also include processed foods that have added ingredients—for example, orange juice **fortified** with calcium and cereals or dairy products fortified with omega-3 fatty acids.

Sales of functional foods reached $35 billion in 2006 and are projected to climb as food manufacturers find ways to infuse more healthful substances in foods.

Although functional foods are increasing in popularity and availability, they tend to be more costly for consumers. They also might not provide forms of or adequate amounts of a nutrient or compound to provide benefits. Additionally, even if a functional food contains enough of a nutrient or compound, it may not be absorbed efficiently.

Functional Components in Foods

Following is an overview of various food components that can provide health benefits when consumed in their original forms or when added to processed and packaged foods.

EXAMPLES OF FUNCTIONAL COMPONENTS*

Class/Components	Source*	Potential Benefit
Carotenoids		
Beta-carotene	Carrots, pumpkin, sweet potatoes, cantaloupe	Neutralizes free radicals, which may damage cells; bolsters cellular antioxidant defenses; can be made into vitamin A in the body
Lutein, zeaxanthin	Kale, collards, spinach, corn, eggs, citrus	May contribute to maintenance of healthy vision
Lycopene	Tomatoes and processed tomato products, watermelon, red/pink grapefruit	May contribute to maintenance of prostate health
Dietary (functional and total) Fiber		
Insoluble fiber	Wheat bran, corn bran, fruit skins	May contribute to maintenance of a healthy digestive tract; may reduce the risk of some types of cancer
Beta glucans**	Oat bran, oatmeal, oat flour, barley, rye	May reduce risk of coronary heart disease (CHD)
Soluble fiber**	Psyllium seed husk, peas, beans, apples, citrus fruit	May reduce risk of CHD and some types of cancer
Whole grains**	Cereal grains, whole oatmeal, wheat bread, brown rice	May reduce risk of CHD, some types of cancer; may contribute to maintenance of healthy blood glucose levels
Fatty Acids		
Monounsaturated fatty acids (MUFAs)**	Tree nuts, olive oil, canola oil	Can reduce risk of CHD

10.3

continues

EXAMPLES OF FUNCTIONAL COMPONENTS* (CONTINUED)

Class/Components	Source*	Potential Benefit
Fatty Acids		
Polyunsaturated fatty acids (PUFAs) omega-3 fatty acids—ALA	Walnuts, flax	Can contribute to maintenance of heart health; may contribute to maintenance of mental and visual function
PUFAs—Omega-3 Fatty acids —DHA/EPA**	Salmon, tuna, marine, and other fish oils	Can reduce risk of CHD; may contribute to maintenance of mental and visual function
Conjugated linoleic acid (CLA)	Beef, lamb, cheese	Some may contribute to maintenance of desirable body composition and healthy immune function
Flavonoids		
Anthocyanins: Cyanidin, Delphinidin, Malvidin	Berries, cherries, red grapes	Bolsters cellular antioxidant defenses; may contribute to maintenance of brain function
Flavanols: Catechins, Epicatechins, Epigallocatechin, Procyanidins	Tea, cocoa, chocolate, apples, grapes	May contribute to maintenance of heart health
Flavonones: Hesperetin, Naringenin	Citrus foods	Neutralize free radicals, which can damage cells; bolster cellular antioxidant defenses
Flavonols: Quercetin, Kaempferol, Isorhamnetin, Myricetin	Onions, apples, tea, broccoli	Neutralize free radicals, which may damage cells; bolster cellular antioxidant defenses
Proantho-cyanidins	Cranberries, cocoa, apples, grapes, strawberries, wine, peanuts, cinnamon	May contribute to maintenance of urinary tract health and heart health

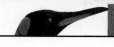

Class/Components	Source*	Potential Benefit
Isothiocyanates		
Sulforaphane	Cauliflower, broccoli, broccoli sprouts, cabbage, kale, horseradish	May enhance detoxification of undesirable compounds; bolsters cellular antioxidant defenses
Minerals		
Calcium**	Sardines (with bones), spinach, yogurt, low-fat dairy products, fortified foods and beverages	May reduce the risk of osteoporosis
Magnesium	Spinach, pumpkin seeds, whole-grain breads and cereals, halibut, Brazil nuts	May contribute to maintenance of normal muscle and nerve function, healthy immune function, and bone health
Potassium**	Potatoes, low-fat dairy products, whole-grain breads and cereals, citrus juices, beans, bananas	In combination with a low-sodium diet, may reduce the risk of high blood pressure and stroke
Selenium	Fish, red meat, grains, garlic, liver, eggs	Neutralizes free radicals, which may damage cells; may contribute to healthy immune function
Phenolic Acids		
Caffeic acid, Ferulic acid	Apples, pears, citrus fruits, some vegetables, coffee	May bolster cellular antioxidant defenses; may contribute to maintenance of healthy vision and heart health
Plant Stanols/Sterols		
Free Stanols/ Sterols**	Corn, soy, wheat, wood oils, fortified foods and beverages	May reduce risk of CHD

10.3

continues

EXAMPLES OF FUNCTIONAL COMPONENTS* (CONTINUED)

Class/Components	Source*	Potential Benefit
Plant Stanols/Sterols		
Stanol/Sterol esters**	Fortified table spreads, stanol ester dietary supplements	May reduce risk of CHD
Polyols		
Sugar alcohols**: Xylitol, Sorbitol, Mannitol, Lactitol, Erythritol	Some chewing gums and other food	May reduce risk of dental caries
Prebiotics		
Inulin, Fructo-oligosaccharides (FOS), Polydextrose	Whole grains, onions, some fruits, garlic, honey, leeks, and and beverages	May improve constipation, promote regularity, gastrointestinal health; may improve calcium absorption
Probiotics		
Yeast, Lactobacilli	Certain yogurts and other cultured dairy and nondairy applications	May improve gastrointestinal health and systemic immunity; benefits are strain-specific
Phytoestrogens		
Isoflavones: Daidzein, Genistein	Soybeans and soy-based foods	May contribute to maintenance of bone health, healthy brain and immune function; for women, may contribute to maintenance of menopausal health
Lignans	Flax, rye, some vegetables	May contribute to maintenance of heart health and healthy immune function
Soy Protein		
Soy protein**	Soybeans and soy-based foods	May reduce risk of CHD

Class/Components	Source*	Potential Benefit
Sulfides/Thiols		
Diallyl sulfide, Allyl methyl trisulfide	Garlic, onions, leeks, scallions	May enhance detoxification of undesirable compounds; may contribute to maintenance of heart health and healthy immune function
Dithiolthiones	Cruciferous vegetables	May enhance detoxification of undesirable compounds; may contribute to maintenance of healthy immune function
Vitamins		
A***	Organ meats, milk, eggs, carrots, sweet potatoes, spinach	May contribute to maintenance of healthy vision, immune function, and bone health; may contribute to cell integrity
B1 (thiamin)	Lentils, peas, long-grain brown rice, Brazil nuts	May contribute to maintenance of mental function; helps regulate metabolism
B2 (riboflavin)	Lean meats, eggs, green leafy vegetables	Helps support cell growth; helps regulate metabolism
B3 (niacin)	Dairy products, poultry, fish, nuts, eggs	Helps support cell growth; helps regulate metabolism
B5 (pantothenic acid)	Organ meats, lobster, soybeans, lentils	Helps regulate metabolism and hormone synthesis
B6 (pyridoxine)	Beans, nuts, meat, legumes, fish, whole grains	May contribute to maintenance of healthy immune function; helps regulate metabolism
B9 (folate)**	Beans, legumes, citrus foods, green leafy vegetables, fortified breads and cereals	May reduce a woman's risk of having a child with a brain or spinal cord defect

10.3

continues

EXAMPLES OF FUNCTIONAL COMPONENTS* (CONTINUED)

Class/Components	Source*	Potential Benefit
Vitamins		
B12 (cobalamin)	Eggs, meat, poultry, milk	May contribute to maintenance of mental function; helps regulate metabolism and supports blood cell formation
Biotin	Liver, salmon, dairy, eggs, oysters	Helps regulate metabolism and hormone synthesis
C	Guava, sweet red/green pepper, kiwi, citrus fruits, strawberries	Neutralizes free radicals, which may damage cells; may contribute to maintenance of bone health and immune function
D	Sunlight, fish, fortified milk	Helps regulate calcium and phosphorus; and cereals contributes to bone health; may contribute to healthy immune function; helps support cell growth
E	Sunflower seeds, almonds, hazelnuts, turnip greens	Neutralizes free radicals, which may damage cells; may contribute to healthy immune function and maintenance of heart health

Examples are not an all-inclusive list.

**** FDA-approved health claim established for component.*

***** Preformed vitamin A is found in foods that come from animals. Provitamin A carotenoids are found in many darkly colored fruits and vegetables and are major sources of vitamin A for vegetarians.*

Source: Originally printed in the 2007–2009 IFIC Foundation Media Guide on Food Safety and Nutrition; www.ific.org/nutrition/functional/#.

WORDS TO GO . . . WORDS TO GO . . . WORDS TO GO

Fortified foods are foods that are infused with nutrients not naturally present in the food in its original state.

10.4 FAT REPLACERS AND SUGAR SUBSTITUTES

Fat Replacers

Low-Calorie Sweeteners

This subchapter covers fat replacers and low-calorie sweeteners (also known as sugar substitutes). An overview of the various types available is provided as an option for consumers who want to reduce their intake of fat, sugar, or sodium.

Fat Replacers

Although fat is a vital nutrient with several important functions, a variety of fat replacers are available to help consumers curb their overall fat intake to lose or manage their weight or to reduce the risk of or manage diet-related diseases and conditions.

◀ SEE ALSO 2.1, *"Functions of Fats"* ▷

◀ SEE ALSO Chapter 8, *"Eat to Beat Disease"* ▷

Fat replacers are designed to mimic the taste and texture of fat. Fat replacers can be carbohydrate-, fat-, or protein-based. Typically, the ingredients used to create a fat replacer depend on how the food product will be eaten or prepared.

The following table outlines fat replacers (as well as their common food sources) that are available to consumers:

Fat Replacers

Protein-Based Fat Replacers

> **Microparticulated protein (Simplesse)**—Reduced-calorie (1–2 calorie/gram) ingredient made from whey protein or milk and egg protein. Digested as a protein. Many applications, including dairy products (for example, ice cream, butter, sour cream, cheese, yogurt), salad dressing, margarine- and mayonnaise-type products, baked goods, coffee creamer, soups, and sauces.

> **Modified whey protein concentrate (Dairy-Lo)**—Controlled thermal denaturation results in a functional protein with fatlike properties. Applications include milk/dairy products (cheese, yogurt, sour cream, and ice cream), baked goods, frostings, salad dressing, and mayonnaise-type products.

10.4

Others (K-Blazer, ULTRA-BAKE, ULTRA-FREEZE, Lita)—For example, a reduced-calorie fat substitute based on egg white and milk proteins. Similar to microparticulated protein but made by a different process. Another example is a reduced-calorie fat replacer derived from a corn protein. Some blends of protein and carbohydrate can be used in frozen desserts and baked goods.

Carbohydrate-Based Fat Replacers

Cellulose (Avicel cellulose gel, Methocel, Solka-Floc)—Various forms are used. One is a noncaloric purified form of cellulose ground to microparticles which, when dispersed, form a network of particles with mouthfeel and flow properties similar to fat. Cellulose can replace some or all of the fat in dairy-type products, sauces, frozen desserts, and salad dressings.

Dextrins (Amylum, N-Oil)—Four calorie/gram fat replacers that can replace all or some of the fat in various products. Food sources include tapioca. Applications include salad dressings, puddings, spreads, dairy-type products, and frozen desserts.

Fiber (Opta, Oat Fiber, Snowite, Ultracel, Z-Trim)—Fiber can provide structural integrity, volume, moisture-holding capacity, adhesiveness, and shelf stability in reduced-fat products. Applications include baked goods, meats, spreads, and extruded products.

Gums (KELCOGEL, KELTROL, Slendid)—Also called hydrophilic colloids or hydrocolloids. Examples include guar gum, gum arabic, locust bean gum, xanthan gum, carrageenan, and pectin. Virtually noncaloric, it provides a thickening, sometimes gelling effect; it can promote a creamy texture. Used in reduced-calorie, fat-free salad dressings and to reduce fat content in other formulated foods, including desserts and processed meats.

Inulin (Raftiline, Fruitafit, Fibruline)—Reduced-calorie (1–1.2 calorie/gram) fat and sugar replacer and fiber and bulking agent extracted from chicory root. Used in yogurt, cheese, frozen desserts, baked goods, icings, fillings, whipped cream, dairy products, fiber supplements, and processed meats.

Maltodextrins (CrystaLean, Lorelite, Lycadex, MALTRIN, PaselliD-LITE, PaselliEXCEL, PaselliSA2, STAR-DRI)—Four calorie/gram gel or powder derived from carbohydrate sources such as corn, potato, wheat, and tapioca. Used as fat replacer, texture modifier, or bulking agent. Applications include baked goods, dairy products, salad dressings, spreads, sauces, frostings, fillings, processed meat, frozen desserts, extruded products, and beverages.

Nu-Trim—A beta-glucan-rich fat replacer made from oat and barley using an extraction process that removes coarse fiber components. The resulting product can be used in foods and beverages such as baked goods, milk, cheese, and ice cream, yielding products that are both reduced fat and high in beta-glucans. (The soluble fiber beta-glucan has been cited as the primary component in oats and barley responsible for beneficial reduction in cardiovascular risk factors.)

Oatrim [Hydrolyzed oat flour] (Beta-Trim, TrimChoice)—A water-soluble form of enzyme-treated oat flour containing beta-glucan soluble fiber and used as a fat replacer and bodying and texturizing ingredient. Reduced calorie (1–4 calories/gram); used in baked goods, fillings and frostings, frozen desserts, dairy beverages, cheese, salad dressings, and processed meats and confections.

Polydextrose (Litesse, Sta-Lite)—Reduced-calorie (1 calorie/gram) fat replacer and bulking agent. Water-soluble polymer of dextrose-containing minor amounts of sorbitol and citric acid. Approved for use in a variety of products including baked goods, chewing gums, confections, salad dressings, frozen dairy desserts, and gelatins and puddings.

Polyols (many brands available)—A group of sweeteners that provide the bulk of sugar, without as many calories as sugar (1.6–3.0 calories per gram, depending on the polyol). Due to their plasticizing and humectant properties, polyols also may be used to replace the bulk of fat in reduced-fat and fat-free products.

Starch and Modified Food Starch (AmaleanI & II, FairnexVA15, & VA20, Instant Stellar, N-Lite, OptaGrade#, PerfectamylAC, AX-1, AX-2, PURE-GEL, STA-SLIM)—Reduced-calorie (1–4 calories/gram as used) fat replacers, bodying agents, and texture modifiers. Can be derived from potato, corn, oat, rice, wheat, or tapioca starches. Can be used together with emulsifiers, proteins, gums, and other modified food starches. Applications include processed meats, salad dressings, baked goods, fillings and frostings, sauces, condiments, frozen desserts, and dairy products.

Z-Trim—A calorie-free fat replacer made from the insoluble fiber from oat, soybean, pea, or rice hulls or corn or wheat bran. It is heat stable and may be used in baked goods (where it can also replace part of the flour), burgers, hot dogs, cheese, ice cream, and yogurt.

#*Appears as corn starch on the ingredient statement; others appear as food starch modified.*

Fat-Based Fat Replacers

Emulsifiers (Dur-Lo, EC-25)—Examples include vegetable oil mono- and diglyceride emulsifiers that can, with water, replace all or part of the shortening content in cake mixes, cookies, icings, and numerous vegetable dairy products. Same caloric value as fat (9 calories/gram), but less is used, resulting in fat and calorie reduction. Sucrose fatty acid esters also can be used for emulsification in products such as those listed previously. Additionally, emulsion systems using soybean oil or milk fat can significantly reduce fat and calories by replacing fat on a one-to-one basis.

Salatrim (Benefat)—Short- and long-chain acid triglyceride molecules. A 5 calorie/gram family of fats that can be adapted for use in confections, baked goods, dairy, and other applications.

10.4

Lipid (Fat/Oil) Analogs:

> **Esterified Propoxylated Glycerol (EPG)****—A reduced-calorie fat replacer. May partially or fully replace fats and oils in all typical consumer and commercial applications, including formulated products, baking, and frying.

> **Olestra (Olean)**—Calorie-free ingredient made from sucrose and edible fats and oils. Not metabolized and not absorbed by the body. Approved by the FDA for use in replacing the fat used to make salty snacks and crackers. Stable under high-heat food applications such as frying. Has the potential for numerous other food applications.

> **Sorbestrin****—Low-calorie, heat-stable, liquid fat substitute composed of fatty acid esters of sorbitol and sorbitol anhydrides. Has approximately 1.5 calories per gram and is suitable for use in all vegetable oil applications including fried foods, salad dressing, mayonnaise, and baked goods.

> * Brand names are shown in parentheses as examples.

> ** May require FDA approval.

> *Source: Calorie Control Council, 2007. Fat Replacers: Food Ingredients for Healthy Eating; Glossary of Fat Replacers; www.caloriecontrol.org/articles-and-video/feature-articles/glossary-of-fat-replacers.*

Low-Calorie Sweeteners

Low-calorie sweeteners—also called non-nutritive sweeteners, artificial sweeteners, or sugar substitutes—provide a sweet taste similar to that of sucrose or table sugar, with few or no calories. They are extremely sweet (often hundreds or thousands of times sweeter than sugar) and are added to diet beverages, yogurt, and other products in very small amounts. They are carefully tested and regulated and have been used safely by consumers for decades.

Currently six low-calorie sweeteners are approved and widely used in the United States. These include (in order of date approved):

- ▶ Saccharin
- ▶ Aspartame
- ▶ Acesulfame potassium (Ace-K)
- ▶ Sucralose
- ▶ Neotame
- ▶ Rebaudioside A (Reb A or rebiana)

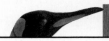

Saccharin

Saccharin, the first approved low-calorie sweetener found in brands including Sweet'N Low, Sweet Twin, and Sugar Twin, contains no calories and is 300 times sweeter than sugar. It passes through the body intact (provides no calories) and is often used in combination with other sweeteners.

Although initially included as a GRAS substance, evidence that saccharin was linked to stomach cancer in rats prompted the FDA to ban saccharin and mandate a warning label on products that contained saccharin. Because later research found no such link in humans, products that contain saccharin no longer have to bear a warning label and it is currently permitted for use under an interim regulation.

Aspartame

Aspartame, found in brands including NutraSweet and Equal, was approved for use in dry foods in 1981, in beverages in 1983, and as a **general purpose sweetener** in 1986. It provides 4 calories per gram (although it's used in such small amounts that it's virtually calorie free), and it is 180 times sweeter than sugar. It is widely used in foods and beverages and provides a taste similar to that of sucrose.

Aspartame, unlike many other low-calorie sweeteners, is metabolized in the human body. It's made of two naturally occurring amino acids: phenylalanine and aspartic acid. It also contains methanol, a naturally occurring substance produced by digestion of other food components. Although methanol in large doses can be harmful, the amounts found in foods are generally too low to cause toxicity (except in the case of some unprofessionally distilled alcoholic beverages).

Aspartame is unstable at high temperatures and therefore cannot be used for baking or cooking unless it's added at the end of the cooking process. Although it has been proven safe for use by the general population, those with phenylketonuria (PKU), a rare hereditary disease, need to restrict their intake of any foods that contain phenylalanine. Foods that contain aspartame must include a warning to those with PKU that the product contains phenylalanine. The ADI for aspartame is 50 mg/kg of body weight per day.

◀ *SEE ALSO 9.2, "Food Additive Sensitivities"* ▶

10.4

Acesulfame Potassium

Acesulfame potassium (Ace-K), found in brands such as Sunett, and Sweet One, has been approved since 1988 and provides 200 times the sweetness of sugar. Ace-K is not broken down by the body and is eliminated unchanged by the kidneys. Potassium salt is usually the substance commercially used.

Although Ace-K contains acetoacetomide—a substance that can be toxic if consumed in large amounts—the amount found in Ace-K–containing beverages is very low. Studies on Ace-K have found no human health problems associated with its consumption, and both the FDA and EFSA confirm its safety. It is approved for general use in foods (usually with other low-calorie sweeteners) such as baked goods, frozen desserts, candies, beverages, cough drops, and breath mints. It is not approved for use in meat or poultry. The ADI is 15 mg/kg body weight per day.

Sucralose

Sucralose, found in the brand Splenda, was first approved in 1998 in 15 types of food and beverages and then as a general-purpose sweetener in 1999. It provides no calories and is 600 times sweeter than sugar. More than 100 safety studies had been done on sucralose prior to its approval, and JECFA, EFSA, and FDA also concluded it's safe for consumers (including diabetics) to consume.

Although sucralose is made from sugar, the human body doesn't recognize it as sugar and does not metabolize it. It is heat stable and can be used for cooking, which makes it more versatile than many other low-calorie sweeteners. It is approved as a general-purpose sweetener and is found in beverages, chewing gum, frozen desserts, gelatins, and other foods. The ADI is 5 mg/kg body weight/day.

◄ SEE ALSO 8.3, "Diabetes" ►

Neotame

Neotame was approved in 2002 as a general-purpose sweetener. It provides 7,000–13,000 times the sweetness of sugar. It is a derivative of a dipeptide made of the amino acids phenylalanine and aspartic acid (two of the same components found in aspartame). From 20 to 30 percent of neotame is absorbed in the gastro-intestinal tract; the rest is converted into compounds that are rapidly excreted by the body.

Prior to its FDA approval, neotame was examined in more than 100 scientific studies, including those with humans where no significant effects were observed. It is also approved for use in several other countries and has received a favorable evaluation by JECFA.

Neotame is heat stable and can be used for cooking and baking. Like other low-calorie sweeteners, it does not contribute to tooth decay. It is approved for use in baked goods, soft drinks, chewing gum, frosting, frozen desserts, jams, jellies, gelatins, puddings, processed fruit and fruit juices, toppings, and syrups. Despite the fact that it contains phenylalanine like aspartame does, a warning statement is not required, possibly because amounts are so small.

Rebaudioside A

Rebaudioside A (Reb A, or Rebiana), found in the brands Truvia and PureVia, was approved in the United States in 2008 and is the newest low-calorie sweetener in the United States. It provides no calories and is 200 times as sweet as sugar. It is purified from the leaf of the stevia plant. In December 2008, the FDA did not object to an expert panel's conclusion that Reb A is generally recognized as safe (GRAS) for use as a general-purpose sweetener. It is heat stable and can therefore be used for cooking and baking.

WORDS TO GO . . .WORDS TO GO . . .WORDS TO GO

General-purpose sweetener is a sweetener that can be used in all categories of foods and beverages.

10.4

10.5 DIETARY SUPPLEMENTS

Definition

Supplement Labels

Tips for Buying Supplements

In this subchapter, dietary supplements are defined. An overview of dietary supplement labels is also provided. Tips to help you make informed, safe decisions if you buy dietary supplements round out the chapter.

Definition

Dietary supplements are products intended to supplement the diet. They're widely available in the United States (and online) and come in many forms, including tablets, capsules, powders, energy bars, and liquids. They're labeled as dietary supplements and include, among others, the following:

▶ Vitamin and mineral products

▶ Botanical or herbal products (may include plant materials, algae, macroscopic fungi, or a combination of these materials)

▶ Amino acid products

▶ Enzyme supplements

Dietary supplements can be made available to consumers without prior proof that they're safe or that the nutrient, health, or other claims they boast on labels are accurate or truthful. They cannot, however, be marketed as treatments or cures for or ways to reduce symptoms of any specific diseases. The FDA does provide safety and other regulations for dietary supplements only after they've hit the market. If a product appears to pose a risk of illness or injury, or if it appears to be adulterated or misbranded, the FDA can take the necessary action to protect consumers, such as requiring it be removed from shelves.

◀ SEE ALSO 10.2, *"Understanding Claims on Food Packages"* ▶

According to the American Dietetic Association's position paper on fortification and dietary supplements, "while consuming a wide variety of foods is the best strategy to promote optimal health and reduce chronic disease risk, additional nutrients that can be provided by fortified foods and/or supplements can help some people meet their nutrition needs."

◀ SEE ALSO 6.1, *"Your Daily Meal Plan"* ▶

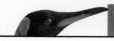

Supplement Labels

Dietary supplements must be labeled with the term "dietary supplement" or with a term that substitutes the word "dietary" with a description of the product's dietary ingredient(s) (for example, "herbal supplement" or "calcium supplement").

The following five statements must be included on a dietary supplement label:

1. A statement of identity (name of the dietary supplement)
2. The net quantity of contents statement (amount of the dietary supplement)
3. The nutrition labeling
4. The ingredient list
5. The name and place of business of the manufacturer, packer, or distributor

Similar to the nutrition facts panel on foods, dietary supplements have a **supplement facts panel,** which lists the serving size, the dietary ingredient(s) and amount per serving, ingredients list, and percent Daily Value (DV) if a DV is available. Amounts of nutrients that do not have a DV can also be included.

Many dietary supplements have a history of being safe. For example, millions of Americans have consumed multivitamins safely. Other supplements that have been safely consumed include

- ▶ Folic acid supplements by women who might be or are already pregnant (taken to reduce the risk of certain birth defects).

- ▶ Vitamin B12 supplements in crystalline form. These are beneficial to people over age 50 who often have a reduced ability to absorb naturally occurring vitamin B12.

- ▶ Vitamin C supplements to help strengthen the immune system. Smokers may also supplement since their needs are higher.

- ▶ Vitamin D if not exposed to ample sunlight and/or don't consume enough vitamin D-rich foods.

- ▶ Calcium supplements to strengthen bones for those who don't consume enough calcium-rich foods in the diet.

◀ SEE ALSO *Chapter 4, "Vitamins"* ▶

◀ SEE ALSO *Chapter 5, "Minerals"* ▶

10.5

Tips for Buying Supplements

If you and a health-care professional (such as a physician or a registered dietitian) decide a dietary supplement is safe and appropriate for you (based on your health status, medical history, and current supplement/medication use), here are some tips to help you make the safest, most informed selections:

▶ Look for a USP logo on the supplement bottle—The United States Pharmacopeia (USP), a nongovernmental, not-for-profit public health organization, sets widely recognized standards for foods, prescription and nonprescription medications, and dietary supplements. These standards can be enforced by the FDA. However, the USP analysis and logo is a voluntary program; if you don't see it, it doesn't mean a product does not meet certain criteria, only that there is no third-party guarantee of that. A "USP™ Mark" on a product label indicates that the supplement meets the following criteria:

1. It contains all the ingredients listed in amounts declared on the bottle; if it doesn't, this could cause a significant health risk, especially for those who take a supplement to prevent a specific health problem.

2. It is pure and free of harmful contaminants such as lead, mercury, pesticides, bacteria, molds, toxins, or other harmful chemicals that can cause health problems.

◀ *SEE ALSO 12.2, "Other Harmful Substances in Food"* ▶

3. It will break down and release the ingredients into the body, where they dissolve; if it doesn't, you won't reap the full potential benefits of the supplement.

4. It has been made under good manufacturing practices (these ensure safe, clean conditions and well-controlled and well-documented manufacturing and monitoring processes).

▶ Be aware that some supplement ingredients, including nutrients and plant components, can be toxic. Some can also be harmful when consumed in high amounts, when taken for a long time, or when used in combination with certain other drugs, substances, or foods.

▶ Never replace a prescription medicine or therapy, or a variety of foods in a healthful diet, with a dietary supplement.

▶ Do not assume that the term "natural" in relation to a dietary supplement means the product is wholesome and safe.

▶ Be wary of dietary supplements hyped in the media—Sound advice should be based on accumulated evidence and not on a single research study.

▶ If you experience any adverse effects associated with a supplement, be sure to contact or see a healthcare professional immediately—Report any adverse effects to the FDA as soon as possible; visit www.cfsan.fda. gov/~dms/ds-rept.html or contact your local FDA District Office (www. cfsan.fda.gov/~dms/district.html).

WORDS TO GO . . .WORDS TO GO . . .WORDS TO GO

A **supplement facts panel** is a clear identity statement that includes the amounts of specific nutrients in vitamin and mineral products and the part of the plant used in herbal products. It also includes suggested serving sizes, information on nutrients present in significant levels, the percent DV when applicable, and other dietary ingredients including botanicals and amino acids (even if no DVs exist for such ingredients).

10.5

11

HEALTHY EATING TIPS

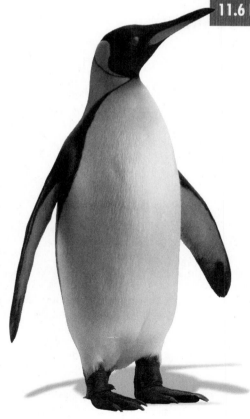

11.1 INCREASING FIBER INTAKE

Increasing Fruits, Vegetables, and Legumes

Increasing Whole Grains

This subchapter includes tips to help you incorporate more fiber-rich foods into your diet. Specific strategies to help you increase intake of fiber-rich fruits, vegetables, legumes, and whole grains are provided.

Increasing Fruits, Vegetables, and Legumes

Fruits, vegetables, and legumes (beans and peas) not only provide a variety of key nutrients, but also are significant sources of fiber in the diet.

◄ *SEE ALSO 1.4, "Dietary Fiber"* ▶

◄ *SEE ALSO 6.3, "Fruits"* ▶

◄ *SEE ALSO 6.4, "Vegetables"* ▶

◄ *SEE ALSO 6.6, "Meat and Beans"* ▶

When shopping for processed or packaged varieties of these foods (which must bear a food label), look for the following terms on food packages to find the most fiber-rich picks:

▶ **Good source of fiber**

▶ **High fiber**

◄ *SEE ALSO 10.2, "Understanding Claims on Food Packages"* ▶

Fruits

Here are some quick tips to help you easily incorporate more fruit into your diet:

▶ Choose fruits that provide a healthy dose of fiber. Some standouts include pears, raspberries, blackberries, oranges, blueberries, and apples. Dried fruits such as dried figs are also a good source of fiber.

▶ Choose fresh fruit over juices as often as possible because the latter don't naturally contain fiber.

▶ Consider 100 percent fruit juices fortified with fiber as an option to incorporate more fiber into your diet; limit these (as with all juices) to $\frac{1}{2}$–1 cup a day to meet your daily quota for fruits or you will overdo calories.

▶ Always keep fresh fruit options available at home and at work. You can keep a small bowl filled with fresh whole fruit (such as bananas, apples, pears, clementines, or oranges) on your kitchen countertop or desk, or keep cut-up fruit or berries in a clear bowl in the refrigerator (or on ice). Restock your options every few days.

▶ Use fresh berries or sliced fruit (such as bananas or strawberries) to top ready-to-eat or hot whole-grain cereals, or add mashed fresh banana, or whole berries (for example blueberries, blackberries, or raspberries) to whole-grain pancake, waffle, or muffin batter.

▶ Top low-fat or nonfat yogurt with sliced strawberries, fresh berries, or pineapple in chunks or crushed; dried fruit such as raisins can also be added but provide less fiber than fresh fruit.

▶ Top salads with slices of green apples, pears, grapefruit, oranges, clementine sections, or halved green or red grapes.

▶ Add banana slices to a peanut butter sandwich (made on whole-grain bread).

▶ For a quick snack or dessert, dip banana or apple slices into peanut or almond butter, bake an apple and top it with cinnamon, make a fruit kebob with fresh pineapple or melon chunks, or dip fruit slices into low-fat or nonfat yogurt.

▶ Freeze grapes or berries to have as standalone snacks or to add to smoothies.

▶ Plop fresh fruit slices into plain water or seltzer for added zing.

▶ As a backup for fresh fruit, stock up on dried fruit or fruit cups (including natural applesauce and canned fruit in its own juice).

Vegetables

Here are some quick tips to help you easily incorporate more vegetables into your diet:

▶ Choose more high-fiber vegetables including split peas, artichokes, Brussels sprouts, winter squash, broccoli, collards, okra, cauliflower, carrots, potatoes, spinach, and mushrooms.

▶ Buy fresh vegetables when possible, but keep on hand frozen and canned versions (preferably without added salt, sugar, or fat) as alternative options.

▶ Keep washed, ready-to-eat vegetables in a clear bowl (to tempt you) in your refrigerator; have them alone or dip them in salsa, low-fat salad dressing, or a low-fat or nonfat yogurt dip.

11.1

▶ Add chopped vegetables (such as mushrooms, peppers, asparagus, onions, or tomatoes) to boost the nutrition and fiber of your scrambled eggs or omelets.

▶ Add canned peas or carrots (unsalted) or frozen broccoli or cauliflower (unsalted) to macaroni and cheese.

▶ Top steamed fresh vegetables with grated Parmesan cheese or melted low-fat cheddar cheese to add flavor and a dose of calcium.

▶ Sauté fresh vegetables with a small amount of olive oil to add taste, texture, vitamin E, and healthy fats.

▶ Top a baked potato with broccoli florets, olive oil, and grated Parmesan cheese.

▶ Make sweet potato French fries, or scoop out the inside of a microwaved sweet potato and add it to whole-grain pancake mix for a boost of fiber and vitamin A.

▶ Start every meal with a vegetable, a small salad with low-fat dressing, or low-sodium vegetable soup.

▶ Fill celery sticks with natural peanut or almond butter and top with dried raisins, cranberries, or apricots.

▶ Add Romaine lettuce leaves and tomato slices to sandwiches.

▶ Top grilled vegetables with tomato sauce, olive oil, or a thin slice of fresh mozzarella cheese, or use stir-fried vegetables to top grilled skinless poultry, fish, or pasta dishes.

▶ Make meatballs or meat loaf with shredded carrots or zucchini, crushed tomatoes, and chopped onions and peppers.

▶ Add puréed vegetables to soups, stews, and whole-grain muffin mixes.

Legumes

Here are some quick tips to help you easily incorporate more legumes into your diet:

▶ Choose fiber-rich legumes (beans and peas) more often; these include navy beans, split peas, lentils, kidney beans, and soybeans.

▶ Use hummus (made of chickpeas) as a dip for raw vegetables, or add it to whole-grain bread and top with cucumbers; you can even use it to top whole-grain crackers.

▶ Add tofu to salad or stir fry dishes.

▶ Make a bean vegetable burger and serve on a whole wheat bun.

▶ Add chickpeas to salads.

▶ Make a chili with kidney or pinto beans and lean ground beef, chicken, or turkey.

▶ Make a fajita or quesadilla with lentils or black beans, shredded low-fat cheddar or jack cheese, lettuce, salsa, and a whole wheat flour tortilla.

▶ Have split pea, lentil, minestrone, or white bean soup as a starter or main meal.

▶ Have baked beans (with no sugar added) as a side dish to chicken or beef.

▶ Mix beans with brown or wild rice as a side dish or main meal.

Increasing Whole Grains

Here are some quick tips to help you easily incorporate more whole grains into your diet:

▶ Choose more high-fiber whole grains. These include barley, bulgur, whole grain wheat flour, whole wheat pasta, raw oat bran, and brown rice.

◀ *SEE ALSO 1.4, "Dietary Fiber"* ▶

▶ Choose more whole-grain foods. These include barley, buckwheat, corn (including whole cornmeal and popcorn), millet, oats (including oatmeal), rice (including brown, colored, and wild), rye, sorghum (or milo), teff, triticale, wheat (including spelt; emmer; faro; Kamut; durum and forms such as bulgur, cracked wheat, and wheatberries).

▶ When reading ingredient lists on food labels, look for one or more of the following as the first ingredient (which are all whole grains) when buying breads, pastas, crackers, cereals, and other grains: whole oats, whole wheat, or whole rye (or any of the other mentioned whole grains).

▶ Don't rely on color to choose a whole-grain product; some breads and other grains are dark in color variety from added molasses or other ingredients, not because they are whole grain.

▶ Have a whole-grain, high-fiber cereal with low-fat milk and fresh fruit slices; if you typically choose a sugary, low-fiber cereal, you can mix $\frac{1}{2}$ cup of that cereal with a healthier one to make the transition easier.

▶ Use crunchy, whole-grain, high-fiber cereal to top low-fat or nonfat yogurt or to mix with dried fruit and nuts for a healthful snack.

▶ Use toasted or untoasted whole wheat breads (including pita), English muffins, buns, and flour tortillas to make sandwiches.

11.1

- ▶ Top whole wheat crackers with natural peanut or almond butter; small slivers of hard, flavorful cheese (such as cheddar); soy butter; or hummus.

- ▶ Top a toasted slice of whole wheat bread or English muffin with a slice of cheese or scrambled egg.

- ▶ Sprinkle wheat germ into low-fat yogurt, salads, or whole-grain pancake or waffle mix.

- ▶ Replace ¼–½ of white flour with oat or whole wheat flour when making muffins, cakes, or cookies.

- ▶ Choose various shapes of whole wheat pasta (for example, penne, fusilli, or macaroni) to make macaroni and cheese, or top them with fresh vegetables lightly sautéed with olive oil.

- ▶ Replace your usual white rice with brown or wild rice and combine with beans or lightly sautéed vegetables.

- ▶ Use toasted, chopped whole wheat bread, cut into cubes, as croutons over salad or to use as a replacement for breadcrumbs to top chicken or fish in baked recipes.

- ▶ Add barley to homemade vegetable soups or bulgur wheat to stir-fry dishes or casseroles.

- ▶ Have air-popped popcorn (with or without some canola oil) or ready-to-eat whole-grain cereal as heart-healthy, fiber-rich snacks.

- ▶ Try some less common whole grains such as amaranth, millet, sorghum, triticale, and quinoa.

WORDS TO GO . . . WORDS TO GO . . . WORDS TO GO

"Good source of fiber" on a food label means the product contains 2.5–4.75 grams of fiber per serving.

"High fiber" on a food label means one serving of the product contains 20 percent or more of the daily value (DV) for fiber (or at least 5 grams).

11.2 DECREASING ADDED SUGAR INTAKE

Overview

Tips to Decrease Added Sugars

This subchapter will help you identify and reduce your intake of added sugars.

Overview

Although they provide energy in the form of calories, added sugars (counted as discretionary calories by MyPyramid and the Dietary Guidelines for Americans) offer few nutrients. Consuming too many foods and beverages high in added sugars can cause excessive calorie intake and may contribute to weight gain. Reducing added sugars in the diet can make room for more healthful foods; promote a more balanced, nutrient-dense diet; and help you lose weight (if overall calorie intake is reduced).

◄ *SEE ALSO 1.2, "Sugars"* ▢

◄ *SEE ALSO 6.9, "Discretionary Calories"* ▢

◄ *SEE ALSO Chapter 7, "Weight Management"* ▢

Tips to Decrease Added Sugars

Here are some quick tips to help you easily reduce your intake of added sugars:

▶ Read nutrition facts labels on processed food and beverage packages to see how many grams of sugar a product contains. Unfortunately, food labels don't distinguish added sugars from natural sugars (such as lactose in milk and fructose in fruit), and both are listed under sugar on nutrition facts panels. You can contact a food manufacturer to see how much added sugar a product contains.

▶ Read ingredient lists on food packages to see whether sugar or any of its aliases is listed among the first few ingredients; if it is, the product is probably high in added sugar. Other terms for sugar include corn sweetener, corn syrup, dextrose, fructose, glucose, high-fructose corn syrup, honey, lactose, maltose, malt syrup, molasses, sucrose, and syrup.

◄ *SEE ALSO 10.1, "Reading Food Labels"* ▢

▶ Look for the term **"sugar-free"** on food packages. Be aware that just because it's sugar-free does not mean it's also calorie-free or low in fat or a healthful food.

11.2

307

◀ SEE ALSO 10.2, *"Understanding Claims on Food Packages"* ▶

▶ Downsize when you drink sugary sodas or fruit beverages; choose a 12-ounce can instead of a 32-ounce cup and save about 250 calories and 65 grams of sugar. Or drink diet soda instead.

▶ Think of sugary drinks as desserts and have them only as occasional treats instead of everyday indulgences. One 12-ounce can of soda has about 150 calories, equivalent to three Oreo cookies or three regular-sized chocolate chip cookies.

▶ When you buy fruity drinks or juices, choose those that say "100 percent fruit juice" on the bottle or can; this indicates the product contains no added sugar. Some 100 percent fruit juice options include orange, cranberry, apple, grape, white grape, and grapefruit juice. Stick to no more than 1 cup per day to leave room for higher-fiber fruit options such as whole fruit.

▶ Swap sugary soda for plain water, seltzer, or club soda mixed with ½ cup of 100 percent fruit juice; this will cut your calories by more than 50 percent and boost your intake of vitamins and minerals. As another option, add fresh fruit or vegetable slices (lemon, lime, or cucumbers can work well) to plain or bubbly water.

▶ Buy canned or frozen fruits with no added sugar and frozen vegetables without sauce; read ingredient lists to check for added sugars.

▶ Flavored foods such as hot cereals (like oatmeal), milks (like chocolate or strawberry milk), and yogurt are often hidden sources of added sugar; they almost always have more calories than plain versions.

▶ Buy cereals, yogurts, and unflavored milks that contain little or no added sugar. To add sweetness, top them with fresh berries, fresh fruit slices, or a packet of an artificial or low-calorie sweetener. Or add a small amount of sugar-free syrup to low-fat or nonfat milk.

▶ Be aware of how much sugar or honey you add to cold beverages (such as lemonade or iced tea) or hot coffee or tea. As an alternative, you can replace sugar or honey with a packet or two of an artificial sweetener or sugar substitute to save calories but still get that sugary taste; you might have to experiment with different ones to find a taste you enjoy.

◀ SEE ALSO 10.4, *"Fat Replacers and Sugar Substitutes"* ▶

WORDS TO GO . . .WORDS TO GO . . .WORDS TO GO

"Sugar-free" on a food package means the product contains less than 0.5 grams of sugar per serving.

11.3 DECREASING SATURATED FAT INTAKE

Overview

Tips to Decrease Saturated Fat

In this subchapter, you learn how to identify sources of saturated fat in the diet and reduce your intake of saturated fats.

Overview

Saturated fats are found in a variety of foods—most notably in animal foods including meats, poultry, fish, dairy products (especially full-fat versions), and some tropical oils and foods made with them. Too much saturated fat in the diet can raise total and LDL (or "bad") cholesterol levels, which can increase the risk for heart disease. Because fat is also energy dense (and supplies more than twice the number of calories per gram than either protein or carbohydrate), too much of any kind can increase overall calorie intake, promote overweight or obesity, and further increase the risk for diet-related diseases and conditions.

◄ SEE ALSO 2.4, *"Saturated Fats"* ▷

◄ SEE ALSO 7.3, *"Overweight and Obesity"* ▷

◄ SEE ALSO Chapter 8, *"Eat to Beat Disease"* ▷

Reducing saturated fats in the diet can save you calories, reduce your risk for heart and other diseases and conditions, and provide more opportunities to incorporate more healthful foods in the diet.

Tips to Decrease Saturated Fat

Here are some quick tips to help you easily reduce your intake of saturated fat:

▶ When comparing products, look for saturated fat listed under total fat on the nutrition facts panels on food packages.

▶ Look for packaged foods that contain the terms **"fat free," "low fat," "low saturated fat,"** or **"reduced fat,"** or that list **"percent fat free"** on their packages.

◄ SEE ALSO 10.1, *"Reading Food Labels"* ▷

◄ SEE ALSO 10.2, *"Understanding Claims on Food Packages"* ▷

11.2

▶ When you choose meats, opt for the leanest cuts ("choice" or "select" meats have less fat than "prime" cuts). The following cuts of beef are considered "lean" or "extra lean" (notice that many have "loin" or "round" in their names): round steak, 95 percent lean/5 percent fat ground beef, chuck shoulder roast, strip steak, tenderloin steak, filet mignon, T-bone steak, eye of round roast, top round steak, bottom round roast, and top sirloin steak. For pork, choose tenderloin, which is very lean.

▶ When making poultry choices, opt for chicken or turkey breast with the skin removed after cooking instead of thighs, legs, and other fattier parts.

▶ Use low- or reduced-fat cheese instead of full-fat options, and use shredded or grated cheese on pasta, salads, and in soups to use less and still get the flavor you're looking for.

▶ If you prefer the taste of full-fat cheese, limit your portion to no more than 2 ounces per day (roughly the amount in two slices). Be sure your other dairy servings that day are low-fat or fat-free.

▶ If you currently consume whole or 2 percent milk with cereal, in coffee or tea, or by the glass, gradually transition to low-fat (1 percent) and eventually (ideally) to skim milk (now often labeled as nonfat). To ease the transition, try mixing a higher-fat milk with a lower-fat one. Or buy a low-fat or skim milk that has nonfat solids and extra protein added and therefore has a more similar texture to higher-fat milks. Some of these milks have "Plus" in the name, such as Skim Plus. Switching from whole milk to 1 percent milk will save you about 3 grams of saturated fat and about 44 calories per cup.

▶ Choose fats and oils that contain less than 2 grams of saturated fat per tablespoon such as liquid and tub margarines, canola, corn, safflower, soybean, and olive oils instead of butter, cream cheese, and sour cream.

▶ Replace some egg yolks with whites to make egg dishes or foods made with eggs.

▶ Use low-fat cooking methods whenever possible; grilled, steamed, baked, broiled, or lightly sautéed options are usually more healthful than fried, battered, or breaded options.

▶ When you're at a restaurant, order foods that are broiled, grilled, baked, or steamed or ask for sautéed dishes made with less oil. If you want sauces or dressings, opt for tomato sauce, balsamic vinegar and olive oil, or honey mustard instead of cheesy, creamy sauces or salad dressings. Order all sauces and dressings on the side; you'll use less if you dip your fork into the sauce before each bite instead of pouring the sauce on your food.

"**Fat free**" on the package means the product contains less than 0.5 grams of fat per serving.

"**Low fat**" on the package means the product contains 3 grams of fat or less per serving.

"**Low saturated fat**" on the package means the product contains 1 gram or less of saturated fat per serving.

"**Reduced fat**" on the package means the product contains 25 percent less fat than the regular version of the product.

"**Percent fat free**" is a claim that can only be made on a "low fat" or "fat free" product. It must accurately reflect the amount of fat found in 100 g of the food. For example, a food that contains 3 grams of fat per 100 grams of food can claim "97 percent fat free" on its package.

11.3

11.4 DECREASING TRANS FAT INTAKE

Overview

Tips to Decrease Trans Fats

This subchapter helps you identify food sources and reduce your overall intake of trans fats.

Overview

Trans fats are abundant in the food supply. Although some occur naturally in animal foods, most of the trans fats Americans consume come from processed and packaged foods and from breaded and fried fast foods. Trans fats are harmful because they raise LDL or "bad" cholesterol levels and can also lower HDL or "good cholesterol" levels; this can increase the risk for heart disease.

◀ SEE ALSO 2.5, *"Trans Fats"* ▶

◀ SEE ALSO 8.1, *"Cardiovascular Disease"* ▶

Cutting back on trans fats can reduce the risk of heart disease and other diet-related diseases and conditions. If it reduces overall calorie intake, it can also promote weight loss or help you manage your weight.

◀ SEE ALSO Chapter 7, *"Weight Management"* ▶

◀ SEE ALSO Chapter 8, *"Eat to Beat Disease"* ▶

Tips to Decrease Trans Fats

Here are some quick tips to help you easily reduce your intake of trans fats:

▶ Read nutrition facts panels and ingredient lists to find trans fats in packaged foods. Choose those that have 0 grams of trans fats and, at the same time, do not have "partially hydrogenated vegetable oil" or "vegetable shortening" listed on the ingredient list. Products are allowed to claim they are **"trans fat free"** or have "zero trans" if they contain less than 0.5 gram of trans fat. But even that much can add up, so avoid partially hydrogenated vegetable oils altogether as much as you can.

◀ SEE ALSO 10.1, *"Reading Food Labels"* ▶

▶ When buying foods that are labeled "trans fat free," double-check the sources of fat listed in the ingredient lists; although many food manufacturers have removed trans fats from their products, they substituted them with saturated fats such as palm oil and palm kernel oil or with interesterified oils listed as "high stearate," "stearic rich" fats, or "interesterified fats." While there is some evidence that vegetable sources of saturated fats are not as much a health risk as saturated fat from animal sources, this is still a controversial area, so you are best off limiting all saturated fats as much as possible.

◀ *SEE ALSO 2.4, "Saturated Fats"* ▶

▶ When you buy processed foods, look for those made with unhydrogenated oils, such as canola, olive, safflower, or sunflower oils, instead of partially hydrogenated oils. Ask for similar items when you go to your local bakery or when you're at a restaurant.

▶ When you buy margarines, choose those that are softer and have more liquid. These are less hydrogenated and contain less trans fat than solid stick margarines.

▶ If you choose fried or breaded foods, baked goods, or other foods high in trans fats, cut your portions in half or save these items for once-in-a-while treats.

WORDS TO GO . . .WORDS TO GO . . .WORDS TO GO

"Trans fat free," which can also be listed as "without trans fats," "no trans fats," or "zero trans fats," on a food package, indicates the product has less than 0.5 grams of trans fat per serving.

11.4

11.5 DECREASING DIETARY CHOLESTEROL INTAKE

Overview

Tips to Decrease Dietary Cholesterol

This subchapter provides tips to help you identify dietary cholesterol and reduce the amount you consume each day.

Overview

Dietary cholesterol is found only in animal foods or foods made with them. Our bodies do not need to derive dietary cholesterol, but many of us consume cholesterol-rich foods, many of which are also high in total fat or saturated fat. Although it's more important to cut saturated and trans fat intake than dietary cholesterol intake, cutting back on foods rich in cholesterol can also help reduce blood cholesterol levels and subsequently reduce your risk of heart disease.

◄ SEE ALSO 2.6, *"Dietary Cholesterol"* ▶

Tips to Decrease Dietary Cholesterol

Here are some quick tips to help you easily reduce your intake of dietary cholesterol:

▶ When you're shopping for groceries, look for items that are labeled **"cholesterol free," "low cholesterol,"** or **"reduced cholesterol."**

◄ SEE ALSO 10.1, *"Reading Food Labels"* ▶

▶ Make egg dishes with egg whites only, or combine a few egg whites with one whole egg (all the cholesterol is found in the yolk). Add fresh vegetables to bulk up scrambled eggs or an omelet. When baking, replace one whole egg with two egg whites.

▶ Choose low-fat and fat-free milks and yogurts instead of higher-fat or full-fat versions; you'll take in less cholesterol and save on total fat, saturated fat, and calories as well.

▶ Instead of solid fats such as butter, consider using vegetable oil spreads enriched with plant stanols/sterols; consuming recommended amounts daily along with a diet low in saturated fat and cholesterol can help you lower your total and LDL cholesterol levels.

◄ SEE ALSO 10.3, *"Functional Foods"* ▶

▶ Replace some meat or dairy meals with protein-rich meat alternatives, including tofu; tempeh; or other soy-based foods, beans, nuts, and seeds.

◀ *SEE ALSO 3.3, "Plant Sources of Protein"* ▶

WORDS TO GO . . . *WORDS TO GO . . . WORDS TO GO*

"Cholesterol free" on a food package means the product contains less than 2 milligrams of cholesterol and 2 grams or less of saturated fat per serving.

"Low cholesterol" on a food package means the product contains 20 or fewer milligrams of cholesterol and 2 grams or less of saturated fat per serving.

"Reduced cholesterol" on a food package means that the product contains at least 25 percent less cholesterol and 2 grams or less of saturated fat per serving.

11.5

11.6 DECREASING SODIUM INTAKE

Overview

Tips to Decrease Sodium

In this subchapter, you learn which foods are rich sources of sodium. You also learn how to curb your sodium intake.

Overview

Although sodium has important functions in the body, most Americans consume significantly more than is needed for optimal health. Too much sodium can contribute to the development of hypertension or high blood pressure in those who are salt-sensitive. High blood pressure raises your risk of heart disease, stroke, heart failure, and kidney disease.

◀ *SEE ALSO 5.2, "Sodium"* ▶

◀ *SEE ALSO 8.2, "Hypertension"* ▶

Too much dietary sodium, when coupled with inadequate calcium intake, can also increase the loss of calcium from bones, which increases the risk of osteoporosis and the possibility of fractures. Excessive sodium intake for those with kidney problems can contribute to edema (swelling in the face, legs, and feet).

◀ *SEE ALSO 8.6, "Osteoporosis"* ▶

Cutting back on sodium can potentially lower blood pressure. Because many high-sodium foods are also high in fat and calories, consuming less sodium (choosing fewer processed, packaged, and restaurant foods) and at the same time choosing more naturally low-sodium options such as fruits and vegetables can help you reduce your overall calorie intake and eat a more healthful, nutrient-dense diet overall.

Tips to Decrease Sodium

Here are some quick tips to help you easily reduce your intake of sodium:

▶ Read nutrition facts panels on food packages to determine how much sodium a food contains. Sodium is listed in milligrams. Look for the terms **"sodium free," "very low sodium," "low sodium," "reduced sodium,"** or **"unsalted," "no salt added,"** or **"without added salt"** on food packages.

◀ SEE ALSO 10.1, *"Reading Food Labels"* ▶

◀ SEE ALSO 10.2, *"Understanding Claims on Food Packages"* ▶

▶ Read the ingredient list on a food package to find sources of sodium in a food product. The following terms indicate the product contains sodium (if listed at or toward the beginning of the ingredient list, then the product contains a lot of sodium): baking powder, baking soda, sodium alginate, sodium citrate, sodium nitrite and nitrate, sodium propionate, sodium sulfite, and soy sauce.

▶ A product that lists 480 mg or more per serving is considered a high-sodium food. Because fast food and other restaurant foods often contain a lot of sodium, seek out nutrition information at the point of purchase and online to help you make more healthful, lower-sodium selections.

▶ Choose fresh poultry and meats over processed ones such as deli meats, sausages, salami, and frankfurters. Be sure to ask the butcher if the poultry or meats are prepared with a salt-containing solution.

▶ Opt for fresh or frozen fish and shellfish over canned or processed forms. You can rinse canned fish such as tuna, salmon, and capers to remove about half the sodium.

▶ Choose more fresh vegetables. If you opt for frozen or canned vegetables, look for those with no added salt and plain versions instead of those made with creamy, cheesy, or other types of sauces.

▶ Use unsalted broths, bouillons, or soups when cooking. To flavor food, add fresh herbs and spices, lemon juice, salt substitutes, or salt-free seasoning mixes instead of table salt. If you add salt to your food, do so after it's cooked; you will use much less (because salt gets diluted in cooking) and still get the salty taste you're looking for.

◀ SEE ALSO 10.4, *"Fat Replacers and Sugar Substitutes"* ▶

▶ Limit portions of condiments such as soy sauce, steak sauce, catsup, mustard, salsa, and Worcestershire sauce to no more than a tablespoon because these tend to be very high in sodium. Pickles, olives, and capers—often used to garnish dishes—are also extremely high in sodium.

▶ At a restaurant or when ordering takeout, opt for grilled, baked, or broiled dishes over fried or breaded options. Ask for sauces and salad dressings on the side and dip with your fork instead of pouring the sauce or dressing over your food.

▶ Salt substitutes can be a healthful option, but many contain potassium; this can be a problem for those who have kidney or other medical problems. Be sure to discuss the safety of sodium supplements with a physician before taking them if you have any medical conditions or are taking any medications.

11.6

"Sodium free" on a food package means the product has less than 5 mg of sodium per serving.

"Very low sodium" on a food package means the product contains 35 mg or less of sodium per serving.

"Low sodium" on a food package means the product has 145 mg or less of sodium per serving.

"Reduced sodium" on a food package means the product has 25 percent less sodium compared with the original product.

"Unsalted," "no salt added," or **"without added salt"** on a food package means the product is processed without salt when salt would normally be used in processing.

12

FOODBORNE ILLNESSES AND FOOD SAFETY

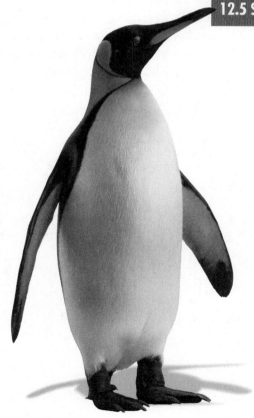

12.1 FOODBORNE PATHOGENS

Overview

Organisms That Cause Foodborne Illnesses

This subchapter covers several microorganisms responsible for many cases of foodborne illness that occur in the United States each year. Symptoms and common food sources associated with each are reviewed.

Overview

Of the 76 million cases of food "poisoning" or foodborne illness estimated by the Federal Centers for Disease Control and Prevention (CDC) to occur each year, only 14 million result from consuming foods contaminated by known microorganisms or microbes, which includes **bacteria, viruses,** and **parasites. Prions** can also cause disease. The other 62 million cases are of unknown causes.

After a person ingests microbes from contaminated food, a delay or incubation period that lasts for hours or days (depending on the organism and the amount consumed) occurs. During incubation, microbes travel from the stomach to the intestine where they attach to cells that line the intestinal walls. Some microbes stay there and produce a toxin that's absorbed into the bloodstream, whereas others travel deeper into body tissues. Although many microbes produce similar symptoms (especially gastrointestinal ones such as nausea, diarrhea, and abdominal cramps), symptoms vary in their onset, duration, and severity; in some cases, they even cause death. Of the estimated 1,800 annual deaths caused by microbes that have been identified, the following three pathogens are believed to be responsible for three-quarters of those deaths:

▶ Salmonella (a bacteria)

▶ *Listeria monocytogenes* (a bacteria)

▶ *Toxoplasma gondii* (a parasite)

◀ SEE ALSO 9.5, *"Food Poisoning"* ▶

These harmful pathogens are particularly dangerous for pregnant women, children, and anyone with a compromised immune system.

◀ SEE ALSO 12.3, *"Preventing Foodborne Illnesses"* ▶

Organisms That Cause Foodborne Illnesses

Here's an overview of some of the more common bacteria, viruses, and parasites that cause foodborne illnesses.

ORGANISMS THAT CAUSE FOODBORNE ILLNESSES IN THE UNITED STATES

Organism/Illness	Food Sources	Symptoms, Onset, and Duration
Bacteria:		
Bacillus/B. cereus	Meats, stews, gravies, vanilla sauce	Symptoms: Abdominal cramps, food poisoning, watery diarrhea, nausea Onset: 10–16 hours after ingestion Duration: 24–48 hours
Campylobacter jejuni/ Campylobacteriosis	Raw/undercooked poultry, unpasteurized milk, contaminated water	Symptoms: Diarrhea, cramps, and vomiting; diarrhea can be bloody Onset: 2–5 days after ingestion Duration: 2–10 days
Clostridium botulinum/ Botulism	Improperly canned foods, especially home-canned vegetables, fermented fish, baked potatoes in aluminum foil, bottled garlic	Symptoms: Vomiting, diarrhea, blurred vision, double vision, difficulty swallowing, muscle weakness; can result in respiratory failure and death Onset: 12–72 hours after ingestion Duration: Variable
E. coli (Escherichia Coli) producing toxin/e. coli infection	Water or food contaminated with human feces	Symptoms: Watery diarrhea, abdominal cramps, some vomiting Onset: 1–3 days after ingestion Duration: 3–7 or more days

continues

12.1

ORGANISMS THAT CAUSE FOODBORNE ILLNESSES
IN THE UNITED STATES (CONTINUED)

Organism/Illness	Food Sources	Symptoms, Onset, and Duration
E. coli O157:H7/ hemorrhagic colitis or e. coli O157:H7 infection	Undercooked beef (especially hamburger), unpasteurized milk and juice, raw fruits and vegetables (such as sprouts) and contaminated water	Symptoms: Severe (often bloody) diarrhea, abdominal pain, and vomiting; usually, little/no fever; more common in children < age 4; can lead to kidney failure Onset: 1–8 days after ingestion Duration: 5–10 days
Listeria monocytogenes/ listeriosis	Unpasteurized milk, soft cheeses made with unpasteurized milk, ready-to-eat deli meats	Symptoms: Fever, muscle aches, and nausea or diarrhea; pregnant women can have mild flulike illness and infection can lead to premature delivery or stillbirth; the elderly or immunocompromised patients can develop a blood infection or a brain infection such as meningitis Onset: 9–48 hours after ingestion for gastrointestinal symptoms, 2–6 weeks for invasive disease Duration: Variable
Salmonella/ salmonellosis	Eggs, poultry, milk, unpasteurized milk or juice, cheese, contaminated raw fruits and vegetables	Symptoms: Diarrhea, fever, abdominal cramps, vomiting Onset: 6–48 hours after ingestion Duration: 4–7 days

Organism/Illness	Food Sources	Symptoms, Onset, and Duration
Shigella/ shigellosis or bacillary dysentery	Raw produce, contaminated drinking water, uncooked foods and cooked foods that are not reheated after contact with an infected food handler	Symptoms: Abdominal cramps, fever, and diarrhea; stools can contain blood and mucus Onset: 4–7 days after ingestion Duration: 24–48 hours
Staphylococcus aureus/ staphylococcal poisoning	Unrefrigerated or improperly refrigerated food meats, potato and egg salads, cream pastries	Symptoms: Sudden onset of severe nausea and vomiting, abdominal cramps, diarrhea, and fever can be present Onset: 1–6 hours after ingestion Duration: 24–48 hours
Vibrio parahaemolyticus/ v. parahaemolyticus infection	Undercooked or raw seafood, such as shellfish	Symptoms: Watery (occasionally bloody) diarrhea, abdominal cramps, nausea, vomiting, fever Onset: 4–96 hours after ingestion Duration: 2–5 days
Vibrio vulnificus/ v. vulnificus infection	Undercooked or raw seafood, such as shellfish (especially oysters)	Symptoms: Vomiting, diarrhea, abdominal pain, bloodborne infection fever, bleeding within the skin, ulcers requiring surgical removal; can be fatal to persons with liver diseases or weakened immune systems Onset: 1–7 days after ingestion Duration: 2–8 days

continues

ORGANISMS THAT CAUSE FOODBORNE ILLNESSES
IN THE UNITED STATES (CONTINUED)

Organism/Illness	Food Sources	Symptoms, Onset, and Duration
Viruses:		
Hepatitis A/ hepatitis	Raw produce, contaminated drinking water, uncooked foods and cooked foods that are not reheated after contact with an infected food handler, shellfish from contaminated waters	Symptoms: Diarrhea, dark urine, jaundice, and flulike symptoms (such as fever, headache, nausea, and abdominal pain) Onset: 28 days average (15–50 days) after ingestion Duration: 2 weeks to 3 months
Noroviruses/ variously called viral gastroenteritis, winter diarrhea, acute nonbacterial gastroenteritis, food poisoning, and food infection	Raw produce, contaminated drinking water, uncooked foods, cooked foods that are not reheated after contact with an infected food handler, shellfish from contaminated waters	Symptoms: Nausea, vomiting, abdominal cramping, diarrhea, fever, headache; diarrhea is more common in adults, vomiting is more common in children Onset: 12–48 hours after ingestion Duration: 12–60 hours
Parasites:		
Anisakis simplex/ Herring worm	Raw or undercooked fish, especially cod, haddock, fluke, Pacific salmon, herring, flounder, and monkfish	Symptoms: Tingling or tickling sensation in throat, acute abdominal pain, nausea Onset: 1 hour to 2 weeks after ingestion Duration: 3 weeks
Cryptosporidium/ intestinal cryptosporidiosis	Uncooked food or food contaminated by an ill food handler after cooking, contaminated drinking water	Symptoms: Diarrhea (usually watery), loss of appetite, substantial weight loss, stomach cramps, nausea, vomiting, fatigue

Organism/Illness	Food Sources	Symptoms, Onset, and Duration
		Onset: 1–14 days, usually at least 1 week Duration: Can be remitting and relapsing over weeks to months
Cyclospora cayetanensis/ cyclosporiasis	Various types of fresh produce (imported berries, lettuce, basil)	Symptoms: Diarrhea (usually watery), loss of appetite, substantial weight loss, stomach cramps, nausea, vomiting, fatigue Onset: 1–14 days, usually at least 1 week Duration: Can be remitting and relapsing over weeks to months
Giardia lamblia/ giardiasis	Water or food contaminated with human feces	Symptoms: Diarrhea, gas or flatulence, greasy stools that tend to float, stomach or abdominal cramps, nausea Onset: 1–2 weeks (average 7 days) after ingestion Duration: 2–6 weeks
Toxoplasma gondii/ toxoplasmosis	Raw or partially cooked meat, especially pork, lamb, or venison	Symptoms: Flulike symptoms (swollen lymph nodes and muscle aches) Onset: 10–13 days Duration: A few days to several weeks

Sources: United States Food and Drug Administration, www.cfsan.fda.gov/~dms/ff15bugs, www.cfsan.fda.gov/~mow/chap25.html; Centers for Disease Control, www.cdc.gov/ncidod/dpd/parasites/ Giardiasis/factsht_giardia.htm, and www.medicinenet.com/toxoplasmosis/article.htm.

Bacteria are single-celled organisms that can exist as free-living organisms or as parasites; they're found in air, soil, the human body, and other places, and many cause diseases or infections.

Viruses are microorganisms that cause many infections and rare diseases. They need to invade and become a part of living cells to grow and reproduce.

Parasites are organisms that cause infections and other health problems. They can't survive on their own, so they depend on other organisms for life and for nourishment.

Prions are proteins found in humans and mammals. When they change shape, they can cause bovine spongiform encephalopathy (BSE), commonly called "mad cow disease." Eating beef contaminated with BSE can cause a variant of Creutzfeldt-Jakob Disease (vCJD) in humans. Body parts of cows that can contain these abnormal proteins are banned from the food supply.

12.2 OTHER HARMFUL SUBSTANCES IN FOOD

Pesticides

Methylmercury

Aflotoxins

Ciguatera

Scombroid Toxin

Acrylamide

Other Chemicals

This subchapter reviews many substances that naturally occur in or are added to foods that can have harmful effects in humans.

Pesticides

Pesticides are substances used to prevent, destroy, or ward off pests (including insects, weeds, mold, fungus, and bacteria) on plants, vegetables, fruits, and animals. Some common pesticides include insecticides, herbicides, fungicides, rodenticides, and antimicrobials.

Although pesticides play an important role in food production, too much exposure over time can have harmful effects, especially in children. Laboratory studies have shown pesticide exposure can cause birth defects, nerve damage, or cancer. They can also block absorption of nutrients and adversely affect growth and development in children.

The Environmental Protection Agency (EPA) sets strict limits for pesticides in foods called tolerances or maximum residue limits (MRLs) to protect consumers from exposure to high levels. The EPA tracks the use of pesticides in foods (including those children typically consume) and the cumulative effect of exposure to pesticides and other chemicals. The FDA analyzes thousands of foods for their pesticide residue levels and, along with the USDA, monitors foods to ensure pesticides are safe and that they meet set limits.

Following are some tips to help you reduce your exposure to pesticides (and make food safer and more healthful, in general).

▶ Wash and scrub all fresh fruits and vegetables thoroughly under running water to help remove bacteria and traces of chemicals and dirt that are on the surface and hidden in crevices.

▶ Peel fruits and vegetables, and discard outer leaves of leafy vegetables to further reduce dirt, bacteria, and pesticides.

▶ Trim visible fat on meats and remove skin from fish and poultry (pesticides collect in fat) before you eat it.

▶ Vary your diet by eating a variety of foods; this will minimize your exposure to harmful chemicals (including pesticides) in food while helping you expand your overall nutrient intake.

◀ SEE ALSO 6.2, *"Your Daily Meal Pattern"* ▷

◀ SEE ALSO 12.3, *"Preventing Foodborne Illnesses"* ▶

To reduce exposure to pesticides and other chemicals, many consumers turn to **organic foods.** Sales in 2008 were expected to reach $24 billion. The Organic Foods Production Act (OFPA) and the National Organic Program (NOP) assure customers that the raw, fresh products and processed ones they buy were produced, processed, handled, and certified to national organic standards. Products can use the terms **"100 percent organic," "organic,"** or **"made with organic ingredients"** if they meet NOP standardized definitions for such terms.

Organic foods contain much fewer pesticides than conventionally grown foods, though they may contain certain pesticides that are natural or approved synthetic versions. But like conventionally grown foods, organic foods are still vulnerable to disease-causing microorganisms. At this time, research is inconclusive about whether organic foods are more healthful or nutritious than conventionally grown foods.

Methylmercury

Mercury is a heavy metal that is near-ubiquitous in our modern environment. It can dissolve in water where bacteria cause chemical changes that convert it to methylmercury, its more toxic form. Nearly all fish and shellfish contain at least trace amounts of methylmercury they absorb from the water and that has accumulated from eating smaller fish that contain the **pollutant.**

Although methylmercury poses little risk for most people, unless they regularly eat a lot of fish, it accumulates in the bloodstream and is especially harmful to certain populations, including pregnant and nursing women, unborn fetuses, infants and young children (whose nervous systems are underdeveloped), and those who are immunocompromised. Effects of overexposure to methylmercury in children can include impaired behavioral and neurological function. Adults can also experience neurological, cardiovascular, or immune-related problems. Symptoms of long-term exposure to methylmercury include:

▶ Impaired vision (such as double vision or problems with peripheral vision) or blindness

▶ Numbness, pain, or other unusual sensations in the hands, in the feet, and around the mouth

▶ Impaired coordination

▶ Inability to walk well

▶ Hearing or speech problems

▶ Muscle weakness

▶ Uncontrollable shaking or tremors

▶ Memory problems

Methylmercury can be eliminated from the body naturally, once the source of excessive intake is removed, but it can take more than a year for high levels to subside to a safe level.

Fish, especially fatty fish, is recommended as part of a healthy balanced diet because it contains high-quality protein, has little saturated fat and cholesterol, and provides DHA and EPA (healthful omega-3 polyunsaturated fats). To help pregnant or nursing women and young children safely consume fish to reap their nutritional and health benefits while minimizing risks associated with exposure to methylmercury, the FDA and the EPA advise the following:

▶ Avoid shark, tilefish, or king mackerel (these contain high levels of methylmercury).

▶ Consume up to 12 ounces each week (an amount equal to four decks of cards) of shrimp, canned light tuna, salmon, pollock, and catfish (these contain low levels of methylmercury).

▶ If you choose canned or fresh albacore or "white" tuna (which contains more methylmercury than light tuna), limit weekly intake to 6 ounces (an amount equal to two decks of cards).

▶ If you eat locally caught fish but don't know how much methylmercury it contains, limit weekly intake to 6 ounces (an amount equal to two decks of cards).

◀ SEE ALSO 2.3, *"Polyunsaturated Fats"* ▶

◀ SEE ALSO 3.3, *"Animal Sources of Protein"* ▶

Those who think they've been exposed to high levels of methylmercury should consult a doctor. Treatment often includes medicines called chelators to remove mercury from the blood and away from the brain and kidneys. These medications must be used for weeks or months.

Aflatoxins

Aflatoxins are poisons produced by mold that can develop at any time during food production, processing, transport, or storage. High heat and humidity or droughts create ideal conditions for the growth of molds that create aflatoxins. Foods most vulnerable to contamination with aflatoxins include

- ▶ Corn and corn products
- ▶ Cottonseed
- ▶ Peanuts and peanut products (such as nut butters)
- ▶ Tree nuts (including Brazil nuts, pecans, pistachio nuts, and walnuts)
- ▶ Milk

Contamination with aflatoxins can cause liver damage or cancer. Although this is more of a problem in undeveloped or developing countries, the FDA has established action levels for aflotoxins found in foods to be consumed by humans or fed to animals (including corn, grains, and other foods) to protect the health of both humans and animals.

It's important to store nuts, grains, and other foods in a sealed, airtight container in a cool, dry place. It's also important to check "Use By" dates on food labels, if provided, to protect against spoilage.

◀ SEE ALSO 10.1, *"Reading Food Labels"* ▶

◀ SEE ALSO 12.4, *"Safe Food Shopping and Storage"* ▶

Ciguatera

Ciguatera is a toxin that accumulates in a variety of warm-water fin fish, including barracuda, snapper, grouper, amberjack, sea bass, and other tropical reef fish. It is produced by specific algae (plant-like substances) that are eaten by small fish; these smaller fish are then consumed by larger fin fish that pass on the toxin to humans. Symptoms typically appear within 6 hours and can include these:

▶ Numbness and tingling (that can spread to the extremities)

▶ Nausea

▶ Vomiting

▶ Diarrhea

▶ Impaired skin sensations

▶ Muscular weakness or pain

▶ Arrhythmia and other cardiovascular symptoms

▶ Reduced blood pressure

▶ Vertigo (lightheadedness)

▶ Itching

▶ Excessive sweating

Although symptoms usually take several days or up to 4 weeks to resolve, in some cases they last for months or years. Although there is no cure for ciguatera poisoning, it is rarely fatal. Treatment includes managing specific symptoms.

Scombroid Toxin

Scombroid poisoning (also known as histamine fish poisoning), caused by the scombroid toxin, is one of the most common fish-related intoxications. Some fish (including bluefin and yellowfin tuna, mackerel, skipjack, and bonito) naturally contain high levels of the amino acid histidine. When these fish begin to spoil because they have not been refrigerated or handled properly, bacteria in them degrade substances in their muscle proteins and chemically convert the histidine into histamine, which then triggers allergylike symptoms.

◀ *SEE ALSO 9.1, "Food Allergies"* ▷

Symptoms of scombroid poisoning occur within an hour of exposure and can include

▶ Tingling or burning feeling (or peppery taste) in the mouth

▶ Facial swelling or flushing

▶ Rash on the upper body

▶ Lowered blood pressure

▶ Headache

▶ Dizziness

▶ Itchy skin

> ▶ Nausea

> ▶ Vomiting

> ▶ Diarrhea

Symptoms can last anywhere from a few hours to several days.

Other fish that have been implicated in scombroid poisoning include bluefish, pink salmon, redfish, yellowtail, marlin, and amberjack.

The scombroid toxin is not destroyed by cooking, but proper refrigeration and cooking fresh fish within a day of purchase can reduce the risk of scombroid poisoning. Antihistamines can be used to treat symptoms should scombroid poisoning occur.

◀ SEE ALSO 12.4, "Safe Food Shopping and Storage" ▶

Acrylamide

Acrylamide is a compound used to make plastic and other products. Studies show this chemical is also created in foods when starches and other carbohydrate-rich foods are overheated during cooking (for example, during frying, baking, or toasting, as with crackers, for example). Although there is no consensus at this time about health risks associated with acrylamide consumption, it is considered a probable carcinogen because it causes cancer in animals. The FDA currently measures acrylamide levels in a broad range of foods and works with the World Health Organization (and other organizations) to evaluate potential health risks of acrylamide and other contaminants. Consumers are encouraged to consume a healthful, balanced diet that's moderate in fried and fatty foods.

Other Chemicals

Polychlorinated biphenyls (PCBs) are manmade compounds that have been widely used since 1929 in electrical equipment (such as transformers). Because they were found to be cancer-causing, PCBs were banned in 1979. Unfortunately, these compounds are incredibly stable and continue to persist in the environment (often in soil, water, and in the air). They also accumulate in plants and animals, including fish (especially larger, older fish). Consuming fish contaminated with PCBs can cause a variety of health problems. The offspring of pregnant women can have lower birth weights, delayed physical development, and learning difficulties. PCBs can also adversely affect the immune system; reproduction; and organs including the skin, stomach, thyroid, kidney, and liver. PCB exposure can also increase cancer risk.

Other chemicals called dioxins are created during industrial processes such as waste incineration and the production of pesticides. Although their use is limited, dioxins persist in the environment and can be toxic when ingested, even at low levels. Dioxins can suppress immune function, reduce fertility, cause birth defects in offspring, cause skin disease, and increase cancer risk. According to the FDA, which reviews dioxins, PCBs, and pesticides as part of its annual Total Diet Study, the greatest source of exposure to dioxins in humans is animal fat. Following the Dietary Guidelines for Americans and using strategies to reduce total fat intake (especially saturated fat found in, among other things, animal foods) can reduce dioxin exposure and help you consume a more healthful diet overall.

◀ *SEE ALSO Chapter 6, "Creating a Daily Meal Plan"* ▶

◀ *SEE ALSO 11.3, "Decreasing Saturated Fat Intake"* ▶

WORDS TO GO . . .WORDS TO GO . . .WORDS TO GO

Organic foods are foods that meet standards set by the National Organic Program (NOP). They're grown and minimally processed without most conventional pesticides, fertilizers made with synthetic ingredients or sewage sludge, bioengineering, or ionizing radiation. Organic meat, poultry, eggs, and dairy products are also free of antibiotics or growth hormones.

"100 percent organic" on a food label means the food contains only organically produced ingredients and processing aids (excluding water and salt). (Processing aids are substances added during processing but removed before the food is packaged; an example would include an anti-caking agent found in a dry seasoning mix.) The product can display this term (as well as the USDA Organic seal) on its package.

"Organic" on a food label means the product contains at least 95 percent organically produced ingredients (excluding water and salt). The product can display this term (as well as the USDA Organic seal) on its package.

"Made with organic ingredients" on a food label means at least 70 percent of the ingredients in the product are organic. Up to three organic ingredients can be listed on the package; however, the USDA Organic seal cannot be displayed.

Pollutants are chemicals found in the air, soil, water, and some foods that can harm health.

12.3 PREVENTING FOODBORNE ILLNESSES

General Population

Special Populations

In this subchapter, you learn four general food safety strategies to help you reduce your risk for developing foodborne illness caused by bacteria and other pathogens. Foods to avoid for special populations are also provided.

General Population

Although it would be next to impossible to prevent all foodborne illnesses, several simple everyday strategies can help you substantially reduce your risk of getting sick from tainted foods and beverages. In their FightBac! program, the Partnership for Food Safety Education (PFSE) recommends four core practices to reduce the risk of developing foodborne illnesses:

▶ Clean—Wash hands and surfaces often.

▶ Separate—Don't cross-contaminate foods, surfaces, or utensils.

▶ Cook—Cook to proper temperatures.

▶ Chill—Refrigerate promptly.

Next we take a closer look at each of the strategies in greater detail.

Clean

Proper handwashing alone is the single most effective strategy for reducing the risk of foodborne illness; it can cut your chances of getting sick by about 50 percent. Hands should be washed thoroughly with warm water and soap for at least 20 seconds (or the amount of time it takes to sing the "happy birthday" song) before and after the following:

▶ Handling food

▶ Using the bathroom

▶ Changing a diaper

▶ Handling pets

Although many consumers opt for antibacterial soaps, there's no evidence that they're more effective than plain soap in removing harmful bacteria. And their use risks giving rise to antibiotic-resistant strains.

In the kitchen, be sure to do the following when preparing food or cleaning up afterwards:

▶ Wash cutting boards, dishes, utensils, and countertops with hot soapy water after preparing each food item and before you go on to the next food.

▶ Consider using paper towels to clean up kitchen surfaces; if you prefer cloth towels or sponges, wash them often in the hot cycle of your washing machine.

Separate

Bacteria can easily be spread by **cross-contamination.** When grocery shopping, make sure to separate raw meat, poultry, seafood, and eggs from other foods in your shopping cart and grocery bags. When you get home, be sure to put those items in a sealed container or plastic bag and place them in your refrigerator or freezer on the bottom shelf. Also make sure egg cartons or holders are clean and not leaking; place those away from other food items as well.

◀ *SEE ALSO 12.4, "Safe Food Shopping and Storage"* ▶

Always wash hands, surfaces, dishes, and utensils with hot soapy water before and after shopping for food and before food preparation. When handling raw meat, poultry, seafood, and eggs, be sure to keep them and their juices away from ready-to-eat foods. Never put cooked foods on surfaces that contained raw meats or other raw foods.

Cook

Cook meats, poultry, fish, and eggs thoroughly. Only a meat thermometer (and not the color of the food) indicates whether meat, poultry, or fish have been cooked sufficiently to kill bacteria. Here are desired cooking temperatures for beef, poultry, and fish:

▶ Roasts and steaks—145° Fahrenheit

▶ Ground beef—160° F

▶ Poultry—165° F (be sure to check the temperature in the innermost part of the thigh and wing and the thickest part of the breast)

▶ Fish—145°F (or until the flesh is opaque and separates easily with a fork)

Thoroughly cooked eggs are not runny; they have firm yolks and whites.

◀ *SEE ALSO 12.5, "Safe Food Preparation and Cooking"* ▶

Cool

It's important to always keep cold foods cold to slow the growth of harmful bacteria. Be sure to refrigerate or freeze meat, poultry, eggs, and other perishables quickly after purchase. The refrigerator temperature should be no more than 40°F, and the refrigerator should not be overstuffed; if it is, cold air won't be able to circulate and the food can be susceptible to bacterial growth (which occurs when the temperature is between 40° and 140°F). You can use an appliance thermometer to confirm the refrigerator stays at 40°F or below. The freezer temperature should be set at 0°F or below.

Raw meat, poultry, eggs, cooked food, or cut fresh fruits or vegetables should never sit at room temperature for more than two hours (or one hour when the temperature is above 90°F) before refrigerating or freezing. If they do, potentially harmful bacteria can multiply at a rapid rate and increase the risk of foodborne illness.

◀ SEE ALSO 9.5, *"Food Poisoning"* ▷

Special Populations

Certain people—including pregnant women and their unborn fetuses, infants and young children with underdeveloped immune systems, older people, and those whose immune systems are compromised in any way because of chronic illness or other factors—are at greater risk not only for developing foodborne illnesses, but also for experiencing serious and sometimes fatal consequences from them.

◀ SEE ALSO 12.1, *"Foodborne Pathogens"* ▷

Those at high risk are advised to avoid (whether at the grocery store, at a restaurant or food on-the-go) the following foods that are more likely to become contaminated with bacteria or organisms and cause foodborne illness:

▶ Raw or undercooked eggs and foods made with them; these include soft-cooked (runny or poached) eggs; **unpasteurized** egg nog, French toast, Caesar salad dressing, hollandaise sauce, some puddings and custards, chocolate mousse, tiramisu, cookie dough, and cake batter

▶ Raw dairy products; these include raw or unpasteurized milk or cheeses and some fresh soft cheeses such as brie, Camembert, blue-veined varieties, and Mexican-style queso fresco

▶ Raw or rare meat or undercooked poultry; this includes raw or rare hamburger, carpaccio (thin shavings of raw beef fillet), beef, and steak tartare

▶ Deli meats and hot dogs (which cannot be cooked thoroughly when they're produced); if you choose to consume them, heat them to an internal temperature of 165°F (steaming hot)

▶ Raw or undercooked shellfish; this includes raw clams, oysters, mussels, and scallops

▶ Raw fish; this includes sushi, sashimi, ceviche, and tuna carpaccio/tartare

▶ Raw sprouts; these include bean, alfalfa, clover, radish, and other sprouts

▶ Unpasteurized fruit and vegetable juices and ciders (if you do choose these, boil them for at least two minutes beforehand)

▶ Refrigerated, canned, or shelf-stable patés (such as liver paté) and meat spreads

▶ Refrigerated smoked seafood; this includes smoked salmon, whitefish, cod, tuna, and mackerel (often labeled as "nova style," "lox," "kippered," "smoked," or "jerky")

▶ Deli salads

WORDS TO GO . . .WORDS TO GO . . .WORDS TO GO

Cross-contamination occurs when a food product becomes contaminated from another source, such as another food, a piece of equipment, or a utensil, or a person. Many cases of foodborne illness are caused by cross-contamination.

Unpasteurized refers to foods that have not been pasteurized (treated with heat to kill pathogens in food).

12.4 SAFE FOOD SHOPPING AND STORAGE

Safe Food Shopping

Safe Storage for Perishable Foods

Safe Storage for Nonperishable Foods

In this subchapter, you learn how to make safer choices when shopping for food. You'll also learn how to safely refrigerate or freeze perishable foods and store nonperishable ones.

Safe Food Shopping

It's important to be aware of food safety when grocery shopping. It's wise to keep some hand wipes or sanitizer in your purse or bag to use to remove any bugs that can have landed on your hands after you've touched a shopping cart or basket and handled a variety of items. Also, be sure to buy perishable foods only if you know you can safely store them in a refrigerator or freezer within 2 hours (including the time they sit in your cart or basket). After the 2-hour mark, bacteria multiply at a rapid rate and your chances for developing a foodborne illness multiplies substantially.

◀ *SEE ALSO 12.1, "Foodborne Pathogens"* ▶

Here are some other tips to help you safely shop for foods:

▶ Make sure the grocery store is clean—If the store smells, the store is dirty or dingy, or you see those who work at the store handling foods unsafely or improperly, you might want to find another place at which to shop.

▶ Buy canned and nonperishable packaged foods first—These should be followed by frozen foods and refrigerated foods; save raw meats, poultry, fish, and eggs for last.

▶ When buying canned or jarred foods, avoid those that are bulging—Avoid dented cans and cracked jars or those with loose lids.

▶ When buying frozen foods, choose those from the back of the freezer case because they're usually the coldest and most frozen—Avoid those with damaged packages or those with visible frost or ice crystals; this indicates the item is either old or has been thawed and refrozen.

▶ When you buy raw meats, poultry, and seafood, make sure they're wrapped in plastic and that their juices are not leaking—Place these in your cart away from produce (especially fruits and vegetables that you'll consume raw) just in case the package is leaking juices.

▶ When you buy dairy foods, choose **pasteurized** versions of milk, yogurt, and cheese—Check the "sell by" or "expiration" dates on food packages. Choose milks sold in cartons instead of clear jugs (these allow light in and cause the destruction of riboflavin as well as causing the milk to spoil more quickly).

▶ When you buy eggs, buy pasteurized eggs—Pasteurized eggs are sold in various forms: in the shell as liquid pasteurized egg products, frozen pasteurized egg products, and powdered egg whites (found in baking section). Make sure fresh eggs are refrigerated, and open the carton to be sure they're clean and unbroken.

▶ When buying produce, buy in season when possible—Avoid produce with mold, bruises, or cuts, and buy only the amount you think you will eat within one week. Make sure any fresh cut produce you buy is refrigerated..

Safe Storage for Perishable Foods

Following are safe food storage times for refrigerated and frozen foods that are **perishable.**

FOOD STORAGE TIMES FOR PERISHABLE FOODS

Product	Refrigerator (40°F)	Freezer (0°F)
Eggs		
Fresh, in shell	3–5 weeks	Don't freeze well
Raw yolks, whites	2–4 days	1 year
Hard-cooked	1 week	Don't freeze well
Liquid pasteurized eggs, egg substitutes		
Opened	3 days	Don't freeze well
Unopened	10 days	1 year
Mayonnaise		
Commercial Refrigerate after opening	2 months	Doesn't freeze well
Deli and Vacuum-Packed Products		
Store-prepared (or homemade) egg, chicken, ham, tuna, macaroni salads	3–5 days	Don't freeze well

continues

FOOD STORAGE TIMES FOR PERISHABLE FOODS (CONTINUED)

Product	Refrigerator (40°F)	Freezer (0°F)
Hot Dogs and Luncheon Meats		
Hot dogs,		
Opened package	1 week	1–2 months
Unopened package	2 weeks	1–2 months
Luncheon meats,		
Opened package	3–5 days	1–2 months
Unopened package	2 weeks	1–2 months
Bacon and Sausage		
Bacon	7 days	1 month
Sausage, raw from chicken, turkey, pork, beef	1–2 days	1–2 months
Smoked breakfast links, patties	7 days	1–2 months
Hard sausage: pepperoni, jerky sticks	2–3 weeks	1–2 months
Summer sausage: labeled "Keep Refrigerated"		
Opened	3 weeks	1–2 months
Unopened	3 months	1–2 months
Ham, Corned Beef		
Corned beef, in pouch with pickling juices	5–7 days	Drained, 1 month
Ham, canned: labeled "Keep Refrigerated"		
Opened	3–5 days	1–2 months
Unopened	6–9 months	Doesn't freeze well
Ham, fully cooked vacuum-sealed at plant, undated, unopened	2 weeks	1–2 months
Ham, fully cooked vacuum-sealed at plant, dated, unopened	"Use by" date on package	1–2 months

Product	Refrigerator (40°F)	Freezer (0°F)
Ham, fully cooked, whole	7 days	1–2 months
Ham, fully cooked, half	3–5 days	1–2 months
Ham, fully cooked, slices	3–4 days	1–2 months
Hamburger, Ground and Stew Meat		
Hamburger and stew meat	1–2 days	3–4 months
Ground turkey, veal, pork, lamb, and mixtures of them	1–2 days	3–4 months
Fresh Beef, Veal, Lamb, Pork		
Steaks	3–5 days	6–12 months
Chops	3–5 days	4–6 months
Roasts	3–5 days	4–12 months
Variety meats: tongue, liver, heart, kidneys, chitterlings	1–2 days	3–4 months
Prestuffed, uncooked pork chops, lamb chops, or chicken breast stuffed with dressing	1 day	Don't freeze well
Soup and Stews		
Vegetable or meat added	3–4 days	2–3 months
Meat Leftovers		
Cooked meat and meat casseroles	3–4 days	2–3 months
Gravy and meat broth	1–2 days	2–3 months

continues

FOOD STORAGE TIMES FOR PERISHABLE FOODS (CONTINUED)

Product	Refrigerator (40°F)	Freezer (0°F)
Fresh Poultry		
Chicken or turkey, whole	1–2 days	1 year
Chicken or turkey, pieces	1–2 days	9 months
Giblets	1–2 days	3–4 months
Cooked Poultry		
Fried chicken	3–4 days	4 months
Cooked poultry casseroles	3–4 days	4–6 months
Pieces, plain	3–4 days	4 months
Pieces covered with broth, gravy	1–2 days	6 months
Chicken nuggets, patties	1–2 days	1–3 months
Pizza		
Pizza	3–4 days	1–2 months
Stuffing		
Stuffing, cooked	3–4 days	1 month
Beverages, Fruit		
Juices in cartons, fruit drinks, punch	3 weeks unopened 7–10 days opened	8–12 months
Dairy		
Butter	1–3 months	6–9 months
Buttermilk	7–14 days	3 months
Cheese, hard (such as cheddar, Swiss)	6 months, unopened 3–4 weeks, opened	6 months
Cheese, soft (such as brie, bel paese)	1 week	6 months
Cottage cheese, ricotta	1 week	Doesn't freeze well
Cream cheese	2 weeks	Doesn't freeze well